PET Imaging in Endocrine Disorders

Guest Editors

STEFANO FANTI, MD

ABASS ALAVI, MD, PhD (Hon)

PET CLINICS

www.pet.theclinics.com

Consulting Editor
ABASS ALAVI, MD, PhD (Hon)

July 2007 • Volume 2 • Number 3

SAUNDERS an imprint of ELSEVIER, Inc.

W.B. SAUNDERS COMPANY
A Division of Elsevier Inc.

1600 John F. Kennedy Boulevard • Suite 1800 • Philadelphia, Pennsylvania 19103-2899

http://www.theclinics.com

PET CLINICS Volume 2, Number 3

July 2007 ISSN 1556-8598, ISBN 10: 1-4160-6091-X, ISBN-13: 978-1-4160-6091-8

Editor: Barton Dudlick

PET Clinics (ISSN 1556-8598) is published quarterly by W.B. Saunders, 360 Park Avenue South, New York, NY 10010-1710. Months of publication are January, April, July, and October. Business and Editorial Offices: 1600 John F. Kennedy Blvd., Suite 1800, Philadelphia, PA 19103-2899. Accounting and Circulation Offices: 6277 Sea Harbor Drive, Orlando, FL 32887-4800. Periodicals postage paid at New York, NY, and additional mailing offices. Subscription prices are USD 175 per year for US individuals, USD 245 per year for US institutions, USD 87 per year for US students and residents, USD 199 per year for Canadian individuals, USD 233 per year for Canadian institutions, USD 199 per year for international individuals, USD 268 per year for international institutions and USD 99 per year for foreign students/residents. To receive student and resident rate, orders must be accompanied by name of affiliated institution, date of term, and the signature of program/residency coordinator on institution letterhead. Orders will be billed at individual rate until proof of status is received. Foreign air speed delivery is included in all Clinics subscription prices. All prices are subject to change without notice. POSTMASTER: Send address changes to PET Clinics, Elsevier Periodicals Customer Service, 6277 Sea Harbor Drive, Orlando, FL 32887-4800. **Customer service: 1-800-654-2452 (US). From outside of the US, call 1-407-563-6020. Fax: 1-407-363-9661. E-mail: JournalsCustomerService-usa@elsevier.com.**

Reprints. For copies of 100 or more of articles in this publication, please contact the Commercial Reprints Department, Elsevier Inc., 360 Park Avenue South, New York, NY 10010-1710. Tel.: 212-633-3812; Fax: 212-462-1935; E-mail: reprints@elsevier.com.

Printed in the United States of America.

Contributors

CONSULTING EDITOR

ABASS ALAVI, MD, PhD (Hon)
Professor, Division of Nuclear Medicine,
Department of Radiology, Hospital of the
University of Pennsylvania, Philadelphia,
Pennsylvania

GUEST EDITORS

STEFANO FANTI, MD
Professor, Department of Nuclear Medicine,
S.Orsola-Malpighi Polyclinic,
University of Bologna, Bologna,
Italy

ABASS ALAVI, MD, PhD (Hon)
Professor, Division of Nuclear Medicine,
Department of Radiology, Hospital of the
University of Pennsylvania, Philadelphia,
Pennsylvania

AUTHORS

ADIL AL-NAHHAS FRCP
Consultant and Chief of Service, Departments
of Nuclear Medicine and Imaging, Hammersmith
Hospital and Imperial College, London,
United Kingdom

ABASS ALAVI, MD, PhD (Hon)
Professor, Division of Nuclear Medicine,
Department of Radiology, Hospital of the
University of Pennsylvania, Philadelphia,
Pennsylvania

VALENTINA AMBROSINI, MD, PhD
Department of Nuclear Medicine and Centre
for PET/CT, Zentralklinik Bad Berka,
Germany

RICHARD P. BAUM, MD, PhD
Department of Nuclear Medicine and
Centre for PET/CT, Zentralklinik Bad Berka,
Germany

WENGEN CHEN, MD, PhD
Division of Nuclear Medicine, Department
of Radiology, Hospital of the University
of Pennsylvania, University of Pennsylvania
School of Medicine, Philadelphia, Pennsylvania

JOEL DUNN, MBBS
Departments of Nuclear Medicine and Imaging,
Hammersmith Hospital and Imperial College,
London, United Kingdom

STEFANO FANTI, MD
Professor, Department of Nuclear Medicine,
S.Orsola-Malpighi Polyclinic, University of
Bologna, Bologna, Italy

GAIA GRASSETTO, MD
Doctor, Department of Nuclear Medicine,
PET Center, 'S. Maria della Misercordia'
Rovigo Hospital, Istituto Oncologico
Veneto (IOV)-IRCCS, Italy

RAVINDER K. GREWAL, MD
Assistant Professor of Radiology, Weill Medical
College of Cornell University; Assistant Attending
Physician, Assistant Member, Division of Nuclear
Medicine, Department of Radiology, Memorial
Sloan-Kettering Cancer Center, New York, New York

MIGUEL HERNANDEZ-PAMPALONI, MD, PhD
Division of Nuclear Medicine, Department
of Radiology, Hospital of the University
of Pennsylvania, Philadelphia, Pennsylvania

SAMEER KHAN, FRCR
Departments of Nuclear Medicine and Imaging,
Hammersmith Hospital and Imperial College,
London, United Kingdom

RAKESH KUMAR, MD
Associate Professor, Department of Nuclear
Medicine, All India Institute of Medical
Sciences, New Delhi, India

STEVEN M. LARSON, MD
Professor of Radiology, Weill Medical College
of Cornell University; Attending Physician
and Chief, Member, Division of Nuclear Medicine,
Department of Radiology, Memorial
Sloan-Kettering Cancer Center, New York,
New York

GEMING LI, MD
Division of Nuclear Medicine, Department
of Radiology, Hospital of the University
of Pennsylvania, University of Pennsylvania
School of Medicine, Philadelphia, Pennsylvania

CLAIRE LLOYD, MRCP
Departments of Nuclear Medicine and Imaging,
Hammersmith Hospital and Imperial College,
London, United Kingdom

MARK LUBBERINK, PhD
Clinical Physicist, Department of Nuclear
Medicine and PET Research, VU University
Medical Centre, Amsterdam, The Netherlands

AYSE MAVI, MD
Division of Nuclear Medicine, Department
of Radiology, Hospital of the University
of Yeditepe, Istanbul, Turkey

CRISTINA NANNI, MD
UO Medicina Nucleare,
Azienda Ospedaliero-Universitaria di Bologna
Policlinico S.Orsola-Malpighi, Bologna, Italy

MOLLY PARSONS, BA
Division of Nuclear Medicine, Department
of Radiology, Hospital of the University of
Pennsylvania, University of Pennsylvania School
of Medicine, Philadelphia, Pennsylvania

KEITH S. PENTLOW, MSc
Physicist, Nuclear Medicine Physics,
Department of Medical Physics,
Memorial Sloan-Kettering Cancer Center,
New York, New York

VIKAS PRASAD, MD
Department of Nuclear Medicine
and Centre for PET/CT,
Zentralklinik Bad Berka,
Germany

DOMENICO RUBELLO, MD
Professor, Department of Nuclear Medicine,
PET Center, 'S. Maria della Misercordia'
Rovigo Hospital, Istituto Oncologico
Veneto (IOV)-IRCCS, Italy

TERESA SZYSZKO, FRCR
Departments of Nuclear Medicine
and Imaging, Hammersmith Hospital
and Imperial College, London

DREW A. TORIGIAN, MD, MA
Department of Radiology, Hospital of the
University of Pennsylvania, University of
Pennsylvania School of Medicine,
Philadelphia, Pennsylvania

MUAMMER URHAN, MD
Department of Nuclear Medicine, GATA
Haydarpasa Training Hospital, Uskudar,
Istanbul, Turkey

ZARNI WIN, FRCR
Departments of Nuclear Medicine
and Imaging, Hammersmith Hospital
and Imperial College, London,
United Kingdom

HONGMING ZHUANG, MD, PhD
Division of Nuclear Medicine,
Department of Radiology, Hospital
of the University of Pennsylvania,
University of Pennsylvania School
of Medicine; The Children's Hospital
of Philadelphia, University of Pennsylvania
School of Medicine, Philadelphia,
Pennsylvania

Contents

Follicular cell-derived differentiated thyroid carcinoma has a fairly good prognosis; however, the probability of recurrence is high, which increases the morbidity and mortality rates significantly. The most common agent used in patients with differentiated carcinoma for both diagnostic and therapeutic purposes is radioiodine; however, it has been reported that thyroid tumor cells lose the ability to take up iodine because of de-differentiation. Positron emission tomography (PET) using 18-F-fluorodeoxyglucose (FDG) has proven useful in patients with differentiated thyroid carcinoma presenting serologic evidence of persistent disease but negative whole-body radioiodine scanning. There is an on-going debate on the role of PET in revealing the malignancy in thyroid nodules preoperatively. As a functional imaging modality, FDG-PET imaging may have some limitations because of its finite spatial resolution, especially in patients with minimal cervical adenopathy or small pulmonary metastasis; however its accuracy may improve using fusion imaging with either computed tomography (PET-CT) or magnetic resonance imaging (PET-MR imaging).

Medullary thyroid carcinoma is a rare tumor of calcitonin-secreting parafollicular C-cells, and it has a poor prognosis compared with follicular cell–derived tumors. Total thyroidectomy is the treatment of choice, and the prognosis is closely related to the stage of the disease at initial diagnosis. It is important to localize the sites of disease precisely for subsequent surgical intervention; however, measurement of calcitonin levels in the blood provides no information about the location of active disease.

Molecular imaging is the visualization, characterization, and measurement of biologic processes at the molecular and cellular levels in human beings and other living systems. In thyroid cancer, this includes imaging iodine transport, which is active in about 80% of well-differentiated thyroid malignancies. Iodine-124 imaging with positron emission tomography (I-124-PET) is ideal for this purpose because PET provides tomographic images with spatial and contrast resolution. Because iodine-131 is the mainstay for therapy in thyroid cancer, and because success or failure of therapy depends on the degree of iodine uptake by the tumor cells, I-124-PET imaging will increasingly act as a surrogate for this treatment. This approach may serve as a model for individualized therapeutic interventions for many other malignant and nonmalignant diseases.

radiopharmaceuticals, especially SMS-R increases in the absence of any specific biochemical marker or clinical parameter for follow-up of patients after therapy (eg peptide receptor radionuclide therapy, surgery, chemoembolisation, etc). New criteria based on molecular, metabolic and morphologic imaging needs to be developed for correct assessment of response to therapy for these slow-growing, solid tumors.

Positron Emission Tomography Imaging and Hyperinsulinism   377

Miguel Hernandez-Pampaloni, Hongming Zhuang, Stefano Fanti, and Abass Alavi

Congenital hyperinsulinism is the most important cause of recurrent hypoglycemia in infancy and can be caused by two different histopathologic lesions, a focal or a diffuse form, based on different molecular abnormalities despite an indistinguishable clinical pattern. The differential diagnosis between the two forms is pivotal because focal disease is potentially curable by selective resection of the pancreatic focus, whereas diffuse forms require a subtotal pancreatectomy. Different conventional imaging modalities and invasive selective arterial calcium stimulation have been used to identify the two forms of the disease. Positron emission tomography imaging is a widely recognized noninvasive modality that is now standard of care for many oncologic processes based on its metabolic and functional capabilities. Based on the properties of L-dihydroxyphenylalanine as a precursor of catecholamines, this paper reviews the current and future potential applications that this technology has in accurately diagnosing the two main forms of congenital hyperinsulinism.

PET and Parathyroid   385

Gaia Grassetto, Abass Alavi, and Domenico Rubello

In parathyroid disease, classical scintigraphic techniques remain the first choice for localizing hyperfunctional parathyroid glands in primary known hyperparathyroidism and in case of secondary, tertiary, and recurrent hyperparathyroidism. When classical scintigraphic techniques are not diagnostic, however, ^{11}C-methionine seems to offer a good imaging alternative.

The Role of CT, MR Imaging, and Ultrasonography in Endocrinology   395

Drew A. Torigian, Geming Li, and Abass Alavi

Many disorders commonly affect various organs of the endocrine system. The nuclear medicine physician and radiologist must be aware of the manifestations of these disorders that may be detected on structural imaging modalities. In this article, we provide a brief review of the advantages and disadvantages of CT, MR imaging, and ultrasonography. We then discuss the role of these structural imaging modalities in the evaluation of disorders affecting the endocrine organs. In particular, we focus our review on imaging evaluation of the pituitary gland, the thyroid gland, the parathyroid glands, and the adrenal gland. Specific examples of some of the disease entities affecting these organs are also reviewed.

Index   409

Pet Clinics

RELATED INTEREST

May 2008
Seminars in Nuclear Medicine
Instrumentation Update

July 2008
Seminars in Nuclear Medicine
Advances in Brain Imaging

THE CLINICS ARE NOW AVAILABLE ONLINE!

Access your subscription at:
www.theclinics.com

Preface

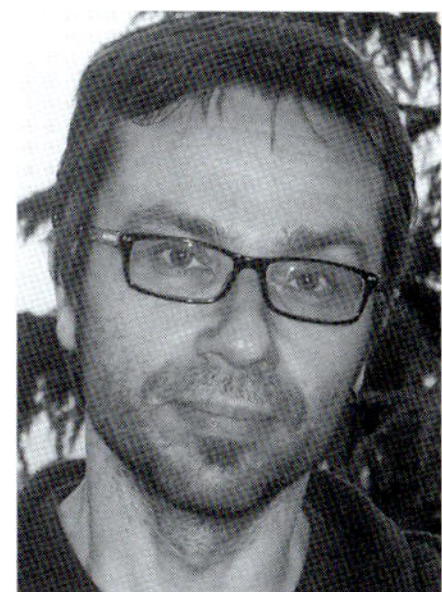

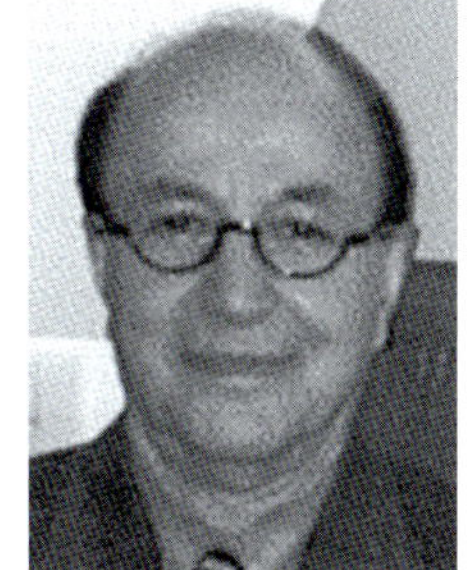

Stefano Fanti, MD   Abass Alavi, MD, PhD (Hon)
Guest Editors

The introduction of 18F-fluorodeoxyglucose (FDG)-positron emission tomography (PET) imaging in 1976 started a new era in medical imaging that has revolutionized and continues to shape the daily practice of medicine in many domains. This is especially true for the investigation of central nervous system disorders, a multitude of malignant diseases, and inflammatory and infectious processes. In particular, the impact of FDG-PET imaging has been extraordinarily strong in the management of patients with cancer. This powerful modality has been quite effective in detecting cancer early on in its course, staging the extent of the disease spread in the regional lymph nodes and distant organs, monitoring response to therapy, and detecting recurrence following treatment. FDG-PET has been useful in malignancies that are aggressive in nature and require substantial interventions to control their growth. Therefore, disease processes that are slow in their course and contain differentiated cells are either negative or mildly positive on FDG-PET images.

Endocrine tumors and disorders are, in general, not as aggressive as tumors of other origins and generally result in chronic disability for the victims affected by this type of disease. Malignancies related to the endocrine system contain cells that are differentiated and therefore have the capability of producing hormones and other substrates. This explains why some endocrine tumors present with symptoms that are caused by the functional activity of the cells contained in these tumors. Therefore, radiotracers that appear to be of importance in imaging this group of neoplastic disorders are substantially different from those that contain undifferentiated malignant cells and take up more specific compounds, such as FDG.

Endocrine disorders have been investigated with conventional single gamma-emitting radiopharmaceutics for several decades. The imaging with these preparations has been carried out using either planar or tomographic techniques (such as single positron emission CT) with some success. The major challenge in developing these techniques has been in developing methods for labeling single-emitting radionuclides, such as iodine, technetium, and indium, to biologically important compounds. A very limited number of such preparations have been introduced over the past three decades. In contrast, the potential of positron-emitting radiopharmaceutics is enormous. Carbon-11, Flourine-18, Iodine-124, and several metallic elements can be readily labeled to biologically important compounds that can be used to image a variety of endocrine tumors. Some elements, such as I-124-NaI, can be used with a minimal preparation effort for examining benign and malignant diseases of the thyroid gland.

Much of the planar radioiodine imaging techniques, either with 123-I or 131-I, can be readily replaced by PET utilizing 124-I[1,2] and tomographic scanning. The element 124-I has a half-life of 4.18 days, which further enhances its efficacy in patients with thyroid cancer where delayed imaging is of great importance.[1–10] Metaiodobenzyl-guanidine and other radioiodine-labeled compounds can be successfully synthesized with 124-I[11,12] instead of 123-I or 131-I, which results in substantial improvement in the efficacy of the performance of this tracer. Certain biomolecules that are cleared slowly from the circulation, such as antibodies and their fragments,[13] can also be labeled with this radionuclide and imaged over an extended period of time. Other compounds, such as carbon 11 (11C) hydroxyephedrine

PET Clin 2 (2008) xi–xiii
doi:10.1016/j.cpet.2008.07.001

(HED)[14–16] or 18F-FluoroDOPA, which provide a high level of accuracy[17–19] in certain neuroendocrine tumors, will be adding a new dimension to imaging endocrine tumors. 11C-HED has also been applied to study the abnormalities of autonomic nervous system of the heart, with promising results.[20–22] Increasingly, Gallium-68 is being utilized to label peptides, such as octreotide, for imaging carcinoid and other similar tumors.[23–27]

For all the reasons enumerated above, we believe that PET will become the standard of care in many disciplines in the field of nuclear medicine, including endocrine disease assessment, and the use of radiolabeled single photon-emitting pharmaceutics will substantially decline over the next decade. We project that the utility of single gamma-emitting radiotracers will be limited to studies where measurement of gross function is the main concern. Therefore, manufacturers of nuclear medicine instruments and the companies that are currently developing and distributing single emitting radiopharmaceutics should diversify their plans to include PET as the main focus for the future markets. Over the next decades, cyclotrons will be the main source of generating radionuclides and will replace Technetium-99m generators at institutions and commercial sites on the global scene. Furthermore, Germanium generates (with a half-life of 9 months) a source for providing Gallium-68 for labeling a variety of compounds that will play a major part in further enhancing the role of PET in many laboratories around the world. Similarly, PET and PET-CT instruments with affordable costs will gradually replace the current planar and tomographic instruments for imaging single emitting radiotracers. In particular, the use of scintillation cameras with sodium iodide crystals for assembling PET instruments should be seriously considered for certain clinical applications, such as bone, cardiac, and brain imaging with PET. This will substantially reduce the costs of performing PET on a routine basis.

Stefano Fanti, MD
Nuclear Medicine, S. Orsola-Malpighi Polyclinic
University of Bologna
Bologna, Italy

Abass Alavi, MD, PhD (Hon)
Department of Radiology
Hospital of the University of Pennsylvania
3400 Spruce Street Philadelphia, PA 19104
USA

E-mail addresses:
stefano.fanti@aosp.bo.it (S. Fanti)
Abass.alavi@uphs.upenn.edu (A. Alavi)

REFERENCES

1. Lambrecht RM, Woodhouse N, Phillips R, et al. Investigational study of iodine-124 with a positron camera. Am J Physiol Imaging 1988;3(4):197–200.
2. Pentlow KS, Graham MC, Lambrecht RM, et al. Quantitative imaging of iodine-124 with PET. J Nucl Med 1996;37(9):1557–62.
3. Frey P, Townsend D, Jeavons A, et al. In vivo imaging of the human thyroid with a positron camera using 124I. Eur J Nucl Med 1985;10(9–10):472–6.
4. Crawford DC, Flower MA, Pratt BE, et al. Thyroid volume measurement in thyrotoxic patients: comparison between ultrasonography and iodine-124 positron emission tomography. Eur J Nucl Med 1997;24(12):1470–8.
5. Eschmann SM, Reischl G, Bilger K, et al. Evaluation of dosimetry of radioiodine therapy in benign and malignant thyroid disorders by means of iodine-124 and PET. Eur J Nucl Med Mol Imaging 2002;29(6):760–7.
6. Ott RJ, Batty V, Webb BS, et al. Measurement of radiation dose to the thyroid using positron emission tomography. Br J Radiol 1987;60(711):245–51.
7. Erdi YE, Macapinlac H, Larson SM, et al. Radiation dose assessment for I-131 therapy of thyroid cancer using I-124 PET imaging. Clin Positron Imaging 1999;2(1):41–6.
8. Freudenberg LS, Antoch G, Jentzen W, et al. Value of (124)I-PET/CT in staging of patients with differentiated thyroid cancer. Eur Radiol 2004;14(11):2092–8.
9. Sgouros G, Kolbert KS, Sheikh A, et al. Patient-specific dosimetry for 131I thyroid cancer therapy using 124I PET and 3-dimensional-internal dosimetry (3D-ID) software. J Nucl Med 2004;45(8):1366–72.
10. Larson SM, Robbins R. Positron emission tomography in thyroid cancer management. Semin Roentgenol 2002;37(2):169–74 [Review].
11. Ott RJ, Tait D, Flower MA, et al. Treatment planning for 131I-mIBG radiotherapy of neural crest tumours using 124I-mIBG positron emission tomography. Br J Radiol 1992;65(777):787–91.
12. Shapiro B. Ten years of experience with MIBG applications and the potential of new radiolabeled peptides: a personal overview and concluding remarks. Q J Nucl Med 1995;39(4 Suppl. 1):150–5.
13. Larson SM, Pentlow KS, Volkow ND, et al. PET scanning of iodine-124-3F9 as an approach to tumor dosimetry during treatment planning for radioimmunotherapy in a child with neuroblastoma. J Nucl Med 1992;33(11):2020–3.
14. Trampal C, Engler H, Juhlin C, et al. Pheochromocytomas: detection with ^{11}C hydroxyephedrine PET. Radiology 2004;230(2):423–8.
15. Mann GN, Link JM, Pham P, et al. [11C]metahydroxyephedrine and [18F]fluorodeoxyglucose positron

emission tomography improve clinical decision making in suspected pheochromocytoma. Ann Surg Oncol 2006;13(2):187–97.

16. Franzius C, Hermann K, Weckesser M, et al. Whole-body PET/CT with 11C-meta-hydroxyephedrine in tumors of the sympathetic nervous system: feasibility study and comparison with 123I-MIBG SPECT/CT. J Nucl Med 2006;47(10):1635–42.

17. Hoegerle S, Nitzsche E, Altehoefer C, et al. Pheochromocytomas: detection with ^{18}F DOPA whole body PET—initial results. Radiology 2002;222:507–12.

18. Pacak K, Eisenhofer G, Carrasquillo JA, et al. 6-[^{18}F] fluorodopamine positron emission tomography (PET) scanning for diagnostic localization of pheochromocytoma. Hypertension 2001;38:6–8.

19. Hoegerle S, Altehoefer C, Ghanem N, et al. Whole-body 18F dopa PET for detection of gastrointestinal carcinoid tumors. Radiology 2001;220(2):373–80.

20. Pietila M, Malminiemi K, Ukkonen H, et al. Reduced myocardial carbon-11 hydroxyephedrine retention is associated with poor prognosis in chronic heart failure. Eur J Nucl Med 2001;28(3):373–6.

21. Nomura Y, Matsunari I, Takamatsu H, et al. Quantitation of cardiac sympathetic innervation in rabbits using 11C-hydroxyephedrine PET: relation to 123I-MIBG uptake. Eur J Nucl Med Mol Imaging 2006;33(8):871–8.

22. Raffel DM, Chen W, Sherman PS, et al. Dependence of cardiac 11C-meta-hydroxyephedrine retention on norepinephrine transporter density. J Nucl Med 2006;47(9):1490–6.

23. Koukouraki S, Strauss LG, Georgoulias V, et al. Evaluation of the pharmacokinetics of 68Ga-DOTATOC in patients with metastatic neuroendocrine tumours scheduled for 90Y-DOTATOC therapy. Eur J Nucl Med Mol Imaging 2006;33(4):460–6.

24. Smith-Jones PM, Stolz B, Bruns C, et al. Gallium-67/gallium-68-[DFO]-octreotide—a potential radiopharmaceutical for PET imaging of somatostatin receptor-positive tumors: synthesis and radiolabeling in vitro and preliminary in vivo studies. J Nucl Med 1994;35(2):317–25.

25. Stolz B, Smith-Jones PM, Albert R, et al. Biological characterisation of [67Ga] or [68Ga] labelled DFO-octreotide (SDZ 216-927) for PET studies of somatostatin receptor positive tumors. Horm Metab Res 1994;26(10):453–9.

26. Henze M, Schuhmacher J, Hipp P, et al. PET imaging of somatostatin receptors using [68GA]DOTA-D-Phe1-Tyr3-octreotide: first results in patients with meningiomas. J Nucl Med 2001;42(7):1053–6.

27. Kowalski J, Henze M, Schuhmacher J, et al. Evaluation of positron emission tomography imaging using [68Ga]-DOTA-D Phe(1)-Tyr(3)-Octreotide in comparison to [111In]-DTPAOC SPECT. First results in patients with neuroendocrine tumors. Mol Imaging Biol 2003;5(1):42–8.

Positron Emission Tomography and Thyroid Cancer

Muammer Urhan, MD[a],*, Ayse Mavi, MD[b], Abass Alavi, MD, PhD[c],
Cristina Nanni, MD[d]

KEYWORDS

- Positron emission tomography
- Differentiated thyroid cancer • 18-F-fluorodeoxyglucose

EPIDEMIOLOGY

Thyroid cancer accounts for 1% to 3% of all human malignancies and has a fairly good prognosis, even in case of distant metastasis if the diseased sites still have the capacity to concentrate radioiodine.[1,2] Papillary and follicular carcinomas are two major categories of follicular cell-derived differentiated thyroid carcinoma (DTC), representing approximately 80% and 15% of thyroid cancers, respectively. The 10-year survival rate of papillary carcinoma is approximately 93% and that of follicular carcinoma is about 85%. Anaplastic carcinoma, the most aggressive thyroid tumor, accounts for about 2% of thyroid cancers and has a 10-year survival rate of only 14%. Medullary carcinoma has its own distinctive histologic and clinical behaviors and is associated with a relatively poor prognosis compared with the other forms of thyroid cancer.

DTC is a disease of the middle and older age groups; it has a peak incidence between 35 and 45 years for the papillary subtype and 45 to 55 years for the follicular subtype. The risk for developing thyroid cancer is known to be increased in patients receiving external-beam radiation to the neck, especially in childhood and in those who have ingested radioisotopes following radioactive fall-out.[3–8] A linear correlation between the dose and the incidence of thyroid cancer was noted with exposures up to 1,500 cGy; however, there is assumed risk at doses as low as 10 cGy. The cancer risk per gray dose exposure is not high at doses over 1,500 cGy, probably because of a killing effect of the absorbed dose; therefore, the incidence of thyroid cancer is not increased in patients receiving high doses of iodine 131 (I-131) for therapeutic purposes.[9] It has been reported that the dietary iodine supply was another factor in the epidemiology of differentiated thyroid carcinoma. There is no overall difference in the incidence of thyroid cancer in inhabitants of countries with low or adequate iodine intake; however, the prevalence of certain subtypes of thyroid cancer varies in these two populations. Countries with low iodine intake show a relative increase in follicular and anaplastic forms of thyroid cancer, whereas papillary thyroid carcinoma is more frequent in countries where iodine ingestion is adequate.[10,11]

Follow-up

The overall prognosis of thyroid cancer is fairly good; however, up to 50% of the patients develop recurrence, mostly in the cervical region, and about 8% of all patients die of the disease. Distant metastasis is encountered in 5% to 10% of

a Department of Nuclear Medicine, GATA Haydarpasa Training Hospital, Uskudar, Istanbul, Turkey
b Division of Nuclear Medicine, Department of Radiology, The Hospital of the University of Yeditepe, Istanbul, Turkey
c Division of Nuclear Medicine, Department of Radiology, Hospital of the University of Pennsylvania, 3400 Spruce Street, 110 Donner Building, Philadelphia, PA 19104, USA
d UO Medicina Nucleare, Azienda Ospedaliero-Universitaria di Bologna Policlinico S.Orsola-Malpighi, Bologna, Italy
* Corresponding author.
E-mail address: urhanm@gmail.com (M. Urhan).

PET Clin 2 (2008) 295–304
doi:10.1016/j.cpet.2008.04.004

patients, most frequently in the first 2 years following initial treatment. The incidence of recurrent thyroid carcinoma increases in cases of incomplete surgery, presence of aggressive histologic subtypes (tall-cell, columnar cell), age greater than 45, large tumor size, and thyroid capsule invasion.

During the surveillance period, the first course of action is measurement of serum thyroglobulin (Tg), a highly specific marker used to monitor the efficiency of initial treatment and detect recurrent and metastatic thyroid carcinoma.[12] However, accuracy of Tg is limited in the presence of antithyroglobulin antibody (ATg) in the circulation. In addition, this test does not provide any information about the disease sites for subsequent surgical interventions. Diagnostic I-131 whole-body scanning is useful in detecting the disease site; however, its sensitivity, especially in detecting small regions, is low, ranging from 42% to 62%.[13–15] It has been reported that I-123 provides optimal imaging characteristics and improves the efficiency of radioiodine scanning, especially in detecting the malignancy in the cervical lymph nodes. However, its limited availability has prevented widespread use of this agent worldwide.[16,17] Moreover, noniodine-avid thyroid tumors are not infrequent because of progressive de-differentiation of the cancer cells and low expression of sodium-iodine symporter proteins during the course of the disease. This can be observed in 10% to 30% of the cases and the incidence rate increases to 40% in the patients at age 65 and over.[18] Radioiodine has a limited role in detecting noniodine-avid tumor sites, despite high serum Tg levels in such patients. Several other functional imaging tracers including Tc-99 m-labeled isonitrile compounds (sestamibi or tetrofosmin), TI-201 chloride and In-111-octreotide have been employed to detect local persistent and distant metastatic thyroid carcinoma. Controversial results have been reported, however, because of patient selection bias and the size of the lesions.[19–22]

In 1930, Warburg[23] reported that malignant cells exhibit an enhanced glucose metabolism. Therefore, glucose analogs can be used to detect the tumor activity in various organs and sites in the body. 18F-Fluorodeoxyglucose (FDG) has been used for detecting malignant lesions in clinical oncology. FDG remains in the cells after phosphorylation to FDG-6-PO4 and accumulates inside the cell over time. Increased glucose metabolism is represented by increased FDG uptake, which can be visualized by modern positron emission tomography (PET) imaging instruments. This allows for the identification of metabolically active sites on PET.[24]

FGD-PET has been employed for various indications in thyroid cancer,[25] as listed below:

Evaluation of the thyroid nodules with or without inconclusive fine needle aspiration (FNA) cytology,

Tumor localization in thyroglobulin-positive, radioiodine-negative patients,

Determination of the extent of disease in high- or low-risk patients,

Prognostic evaluation,

Assessment of treatment response,

Evaluation and management of Hurtle cell carcinoma,

Selection of patients for investigational therapies,

Determination of extent and relationship of the known metastases to vital structures.

FDG-PET IN THYROID NODULES

Thyroid carcinoma is relatively rare among all human cancers; however, it is the most frequent endocrine malignancy, accounting for about 5% of all thyroid nodules.[26] Ultrasonographic (US) evaluation of the thyroid gland has a well-established role in detecting thyroid nodules with its high resolution and availability. The accuracy of US can be improved upon by including FNA in conjunction with this examination.[27] In approximately 20% of the cases, cytologic findings are inconclusive, but eventually the histopathologic examination reveals a benign process in the majority of these cases. Investigational molecular diagnostic tests offer promising results in the differential diagnosis, but they are not currently available for routine application and final diagnosis can only be achieved by thyroid surgery.

The clinical role of FDG-PET in preoperative investigation of thyroid nodules and in differentiating between benign and malignant lesions is controversial. Some studies report incidental focal FDG uptake in approximately 2% of all patients, and in about one-third of these cases the diagnosis is proven to be thyroid cancer.[28–31] In the 1990s, it was first suggested that FDG-PET might be useful in characterizing thyroid nodules and detecting lymph node metastasis because FDG uptake is greater in malignant lesions than in benign thyroid nodules.[32–35] According to some investigators, unnecessary surgery could be reduced by 66% using the information provided by FDG-PET imaging.[36] However, benign lesions also concentrate FDG. In a study by Kim and colleagues,[37] 21 of 36 FDG-positive follicular lesions were of benign etiology, which was proven by histology. In addition, there was no difference between the maximum standardized uptake value of the benign and malignant thyroid nodules. In another study by Kresnik and colleagues,[38] FDG-PET was unable to detect malignant tumors accurately. However, it was useful in referring patients with inconclusive findings to surgery if malignancy could not be excluded. The data reported in the literature so far are not entirely convincing and FDG-PET is not routinely used in daily clinical practice in characterizing thyroid nodules.

FDG-PET IN RECURRENT THYROID CARCINOMA

The utility of FDG-PET has been investigated in numerous studies since Joensuu and colleagues first described FDG uptake in thyroid cancer metastases (**Table 1**).[12,14,39–58] The overall sensitivity and specificity of FDG-PET in localizing the recurrent or metastatic disease varies widely, ranging from 45% to 100% and from 42% to 90%, respectively. The greatest interest has been in Tg-positive and iodine-negative patients. In a large cohort study including 222 subjects, Grunwald and colleagues[41] reported that the sensitivity of FDG-PET was 75% for the whole population, but it increased to 85% for subjects with a negative radioiodine scan. In another study by Dietlein and colleagues,[14] the sensitivity of I-131 whole-body scintigraphy (WBS) was found to be 61%, while the sensitivity of FGD-PET in subjects with negative I-131 WBS was 82%. Based on the data in the literature, an inverse relationship between enhanced glucose metabolism and iodine uptake has been noted and FDG-PET is assumed to be positive in thyroid cancers with low iodine-avid recurrent or metastatic disease (**Fig. 1**). Some patients exhibit different degrees of radioiodine and FDG uptake because of tumor heterogeneity, even in the same patient; thus, the sensitivity of combined radioiodine and FDG-PET scanning

Table 1
The updated list of the studies in the literature investigating the clinical role of FDG-PET in differentiated thyroid carcinoma, including a group of patients of 20 and over

Author	No. Pts	Inclusion	Sens.%	Spe.%	Confirmation
Feine[40]	41	F/U	70	—	Histology, CI
Dietlein[14]	58	F/U	50	NA	Histology, CI
Subgroup		RIS (−)	82		
Grunwald[41]	222	F/U	75	90	Histology, CI
Subgroup		RIS (−)	85	90	
Chung[12]	54	F/U −N	93.9	95.2	Histology
Wang[42]	37	F/U −N	70	76.5	Histology, CI
Frilling,[43] 2001	24	High Tg–N	94.6	25	Histology, CI
Shiga[44]	32	F/U −N	47	NA	Histology, CI
Yeo[45]	22	Rec?	80	83	Histology
Schluter[46]	64	Tg–N	69.4	41.7	Histology, CI
Helal[47]	37	High Tg–N	76	NA	Histology, CI
Plotkin[a,48]	35	NA	92	80	Histology
Sarlis[49]	21	Tg–rec?	67.6	NA	Histology
Chen[50]	23	High Tg–N	87	NA	Histology
Hung[51]	20	High Tg–N	85	NA	CI
Gabriel[52]	54	HighTg–rec?	87.5	50	CI
Nahas[53]	33	HighTg–RIS(−)	66	100	Histology, CI
Pryma[55]	44	Hurtle-cell	95.8	95	Histology, CI, F/U
Shammas[b,55], 2007	61	High Tg–Rec?	68.4	82.4	Histology, CI
Salvatore[b,56]	45	High Tg	71	NA	CI (RIS)
Iagaru[b,57]	98	High Tg	88.6	89.3	Histology, CI
Zoller[b,58]	47	HighTg–Rec?	74	NA	Histology, CI

Abbreviations: CI, conventional imaging; CT, computerized tomography; F/U, follow-up; N, normal; rec?, suspected recurrence; RIS, radioiodine scanning; US, ultrasound.
[a] Pooled data.
[b] PET/CT.

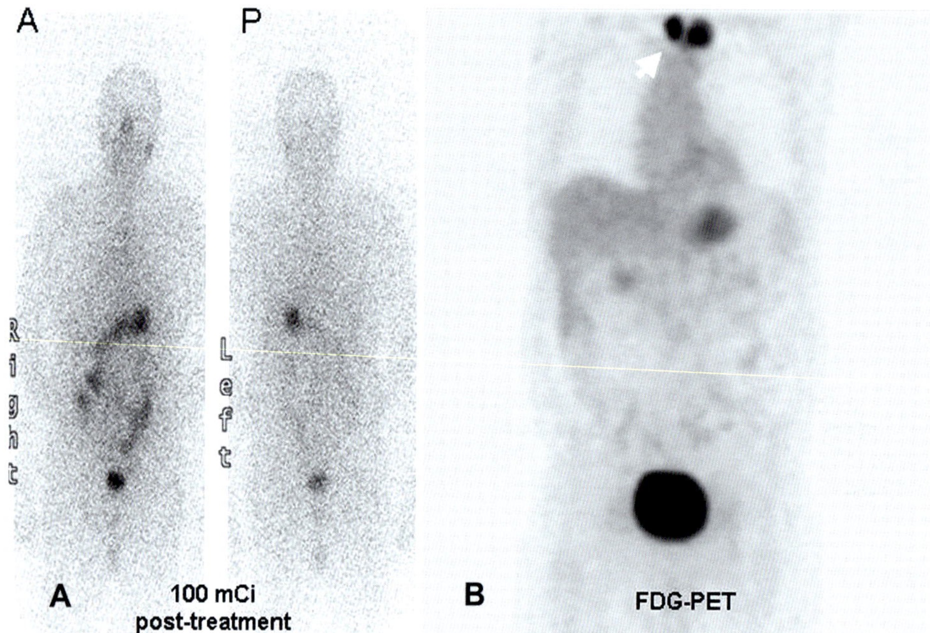

Fig. 1. Posttreatment scanning 7 days after oral administration of 100 mCi I-131 was negative (*A*); however, FDG-avid foci recurrent tumor noted in thyroid bed (*white arrowhead*) proved to be papillary thyroid cancer with histopathology (*B*).

appears to be higher than that of each procedure alone.[40]

FDG-PET is preferred over radioiodine when the tumor cells are known to have low iodine uptake, such as in Hurtle-cell and undifferentiated (anaplastic) thyroid tumors. Hurtle-cell carcinoma has a worse prognosis, compared with papillary and follicular thyroid cancers, and presents unique clinical features, such as higher incidence of distant metastasis and a relatively aggressive clinical course.[59–61] The patients with Hurtle-cell thyroid carcinoma are usually monitored with sequential serum Tg measurements, because more than 80% of the patients have noniodine-avid tumor and the clinical utility of radioiodine is limited in this population. Interestingly, FDG uptake by Hurtle-cell cancer cells is high and PET has a sensitivity, specificity, positive-negative predictive value, and accuracy of 92%, 80%, 92% to 80%, and 89%, respectively, reported in a meta-analysis by Plotkin and colleagues.[48] In another study by Pryma and colleagues,[54] it was reported that FDG-PET had an excellent sensitivity (95.8%) in localizing the disease sites and providing additional prognostic information in a cohort study of 44 subjects with Hurtle-cell thyroid cancer. The localization information provided by PET is extremely important for subsequent interventional surgery or external radiation treatment, whereas the patients would get no benefit from high dose I-131 treatment.

Anaplastic thyroid carcinoma (ATC), the most aggressive thyroid tumor, accounts for less than 2% of all thyroid malignancies and usually occurs in the elderly. It has a distinct behavior compared with other forms of follicular cell-derived differentiated thyroid cancers. Its prognosis is poor, and the patients usually die of local symptoms. Tumor is not iodine avid and secretes no Tg, but its affinity for FDG is reasonably high. The role of FGD-PET in the initial evaluation of these patients is limited. However, in a few studies, it was reported that FDG-PET localized the tumor sites successfully in patients with recurrent ATC (**Fig. 2**).[62,63]

THE PROGNOSTIC ROLE OF FDG-PET

FDG-PET scanning is more likely to be positive as the serum Tg level rises, which is likely related to the volume of the functioning tumor. In a group of 118 patients, Schlutter and colleagues[46] reported that FDG-PET was true-positive in 11%, 50%, 80%, 63%, and 93% of those with serum Tg of less than 10 ng/mL, 10 ng/mL to 20 ng/mL, 20 ng/mL to 50 ng/mL, 50 ng/mL to 100 ng/mL, and greater than 100 ng/mL, respectively. It has been reported that the potential for a positive FDG-PET was higher in patients with a Tg value of greater than 10 ng/mL, regardless of radioiodine whole-body scan findings or serum thyroid stimulating hormone (TSH) levels, although there is no cut-off value defined.[53] Shammas and

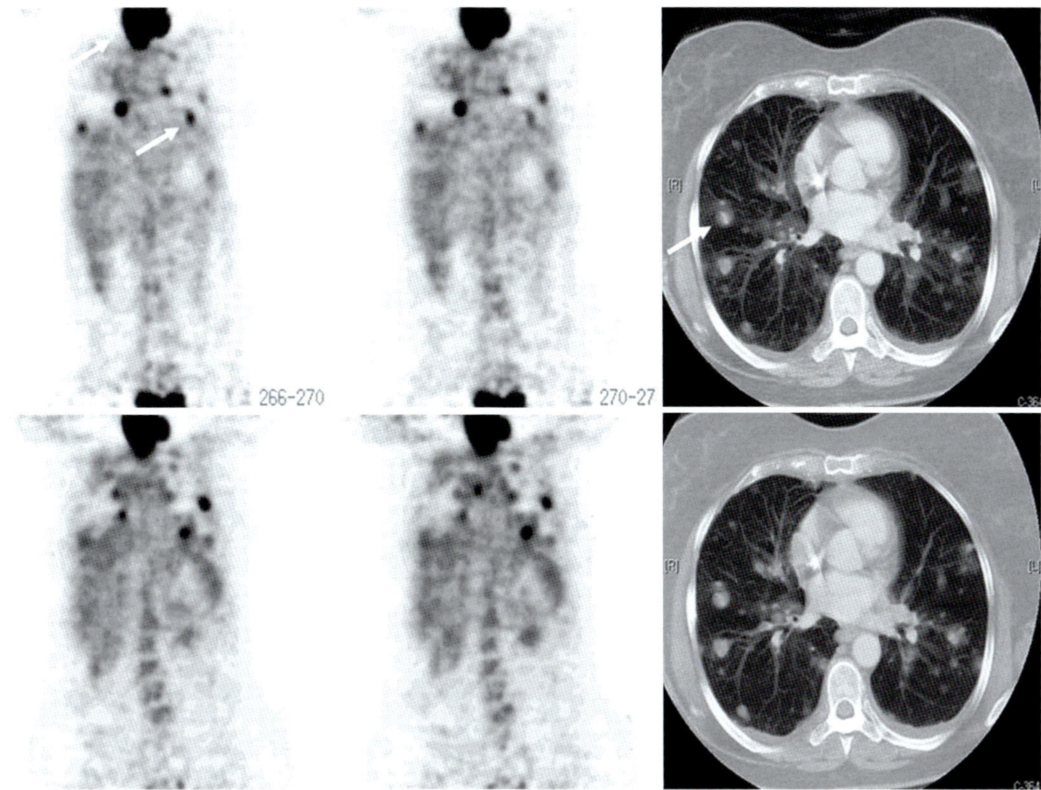

Fig. 2. FDG-PET revealed numerous metastases in the lungs and huge residual tumor in the neck in a patient with anaplastic thyroid carcinoma. The patient had already undergone a conservative surgery previously to ease the neck, as most patients with similar diagnosis died of local symptoms, such as invasion of the major vasculature in the neck or tracheal compression.

colleagues[55] also found a correlation between the degree of FDG uptake seen on FDG-PET scans and the level of Tg in the blood and reported similar findings. In another study, average serum Tg was found to average 293 ng/mL in thyroid cancer patients with a positive FDG-PET scan, while it averaged 30 ng/mL in FDG-PET negative patients.[64]

FDG-PET provides not only localization but also prognostic information about differentiated thyroid cancer, and identifies the patients at higher risk of recurrence and metastatic disease. Wang and colleagues[65] reported that the volume of the FDG-avid tumor was the strongest predictor of short term survival, and the majority of the patients (80%) with greater than 125 mL expired in a period of less than 41 months. In addition to defining the anatomic location and the volume of the tumor, there are some studies which suggest that semi-quantitative analysis of FDG uptake (standardized uptake value) of the metastatic foci is also a prognostic indicator. Schonberger and colleagues[66] have shown that increased glucose transporter-1 gene expression, which is responsible for enhanced FDG uptake by the tumor cells, reflects

an aggressive clinical course and unfavorable prognosis.

FDG-PET has an impact on patient management by localizing the disease site and providing information about the potential clinical behavior of the tumor cells.[47,67] Lowe and colleagues[68] reported that FGD-PET showed more extensive disease than that seen by other imaging modalities, including CT, radioiodine whole-body scanning, and US in 5 out of 12 Hurtle-cell carcinoma patients, and lead to a change in their management. PET findings are useful, especially for leading patients to surgical intervention for treatment.[69,70]

Recently, there has been a debate about the use of recombinant human thyrotropin (rhTSH) to improve the sensitivity of FDG-PET imaging in detecting the persistent differentiated thyroid carcinoma. It is also recommended to use rhTSH in patients who are unable to tolerate the side effects of long-term hypothyroidism or generate elevated endogenous rhTSH levels for radioiodine treatment.[35,71] According to some investigators, rhTSH stimulates cellular metabolism in thyroid cells; therefore, the accuracy of FDG-PET imaging may be higher than that of serum Tg levels and radioiodine whole-body scanning.[72–76] Generally, the sensitivity of FDG-PET is higher when performed during rhTSH stimulation rather than during rhTSH suppression, and it is reported in several studies that more FDG-avid lesion sites are seen with rhTSH stimulation than with rhTSH suppression,[77–80] while in some others no significant difference on scan interpretation is noted.[42] The decision to use rhTSH in clinical practice should take into account the potential benefits and the cost of the agent, especially in patients with elevated serum Tg levels and iodine-negative scan findings.

THE POTENTIALS AND PITFALLS
Non-FDG-PET Imaging in Thyroid Cancer

The clinical utility of PET will improve in detecting recurrent and metastatic thyroid carcinoma as more sensitive and specific tracers other than FDG are introduced in the future. One example is I-124, a cyclotron-produced isotope with a half-life of 4.2 days that has been used for dosimetry purposes in thyroid cancer patients.[81–83] I-124 has several other favorable features. It offers superior imaging characteristics, compared with I-131 and I-123, and a PET study can be performed as early as 24 hours after injection, enabling timely management of patients. Moreover, it delivers a negligible radiation dose to the functional thyroid cells and avoids unnecessary exposure to adjacent tissues. However, limited availability restricts the widespread use of I-124 in routine clinical practice.

Role of Correlative Imaging

Recurrence in the thyroid bed and metastasis to the cervical node are common with thyroid cancer, especially in patients with papillary carcinoma. In the literature, the clinical role of FDG-PET in detecting lymph node metastasis has been defined at primary staging and in the surveillance period.[84] The contrast resolution of PET has been reported to be excellent as a functional imaging modality but it is still low when compared with anatomic imaging; therefore, a negative PET does not exclude malignancy. US is the predominant method for the evaluation of the head and neck region because it reveals lesions as small as 2 mm to 3 mm with high-resolution phase array transducers, and provides detailed anatomic and physiologic information with advanced technologies, such as color flow and power Doppler. It was reported that the sensitivity and specificity of US ranged from 95.3% to 100% and 70% to 85.7%, respectively.[43,85] US-guided FNA cytology from the suspicious lesions is a fast and accurate procedure for establishing a definitive diagnosis.[28,38] FDG-PET, along with US, was also useful in discriminating between the persistent tumor and nonspecific changes in the postsurgical neck region because of relatively high physiologic uptake of FDG in complex structures of the pharynx, larynx, and muscles of the lateral neck. Coregistered PET and CT/MR imaging images improve the diagnosis of metastatic foci by providing metabolic information and by precise anatomic localization of the tumor (**Fig. 3**). In a study by Palmedo and colleagues,[86] PET images obtained from 40 subjects

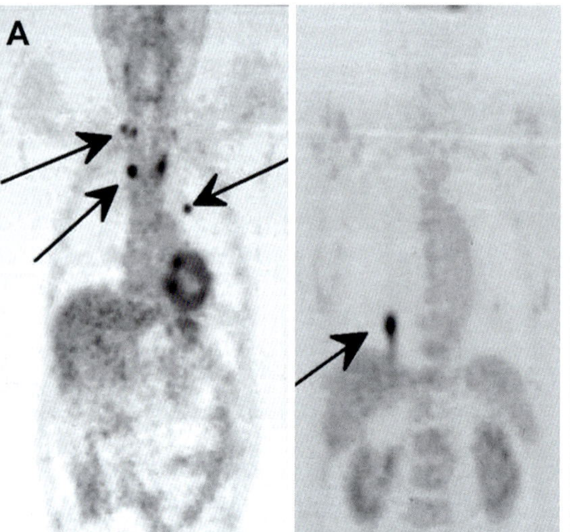
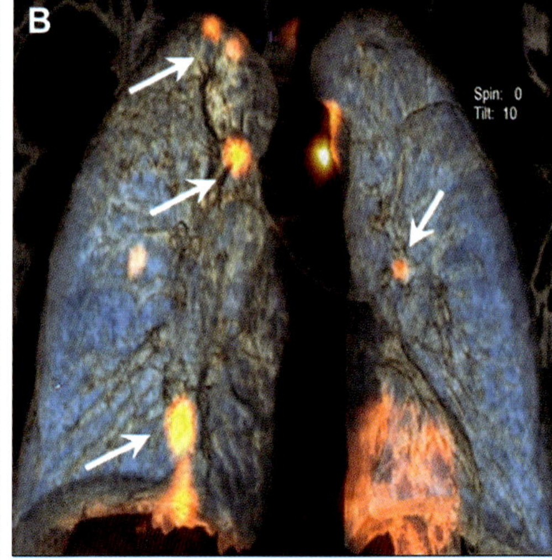

Fig. 3. Integrated anatomic imaging with CT contributes to establish a definitive diagnosis, providing precise anatomic localization and metabolic status of the lesions. FDG-avid lesions (*black arrows*) in the mediastinum and the lungs (*A*) were fused on a three dimensional CT image in the patient above (*B*) with metastatic papillary carcinoma (*white arrows*).

with elevated Tg levels were evaluated alone and fused with a CT map. It was reported that PET and PET/CT had an accuracy of 78% and 93%, respectively. Thus, it is clear that integrated PET/CT devices using sequential acquisition of structural and metabolic information for one session will be of value for accurate localization of the diseased sites, as stated in several other reports.[57,58,87]

Small metastatic lesions in the lungs, as well as minimal cervical adenopathy, pose problems of false-negative PET results. Ilgan and colleagues[88] reported that high-resolution computerized tomography was useful in detecting small metastatic deposits in the lungs. Even in cases of proven cervical lymph node metastasis, a spiral CT is recommended to exclude the metastatic disease in the lungs in patients presenting with high serum Tg levels before planning cervical dissection. On the other hand, PET/CT is useful in discriminating nonspecific FDG uptake from malignant lesions not only in the head and neck region, but also in the lungs and bone marrow. Nakamoto and colleagues[89,90] reported that CT improved the diagnostic ability of FDG-PET by reducing the false-positive findings for bone marrow involvement. To date, controversial results were obtained on the role of FDG-PET in detecting osseous metastasis in patients with differentiated thyroid carcinoma in several studies. It was reported that FDG-PET failed to reveal bone marrow metastasis, possibly because of low degree malignancy of this tumor, as the diseased site exhibited radioiodine uptake. On the other hand, Schirrmeister and colleagues,[40,91] suggested that 18-Fluorine PET was more sensitive than radionuclide bone scanning in patients with differentiated thyroid carcinoma.

SUMMARY

The mortality of differentiated thyroid carcinoma is one of the lowest in all human cancers. However, the morbidity, because of recurrent or metastatic disease, is still high. Established tests allow prompt treatment and follow-up of high-risk patients who are most likely to develop a recurrence and also would reduce the morbidity and mortality from this cancer. Radioiodine is the major agent for diagnostic and therapeutic purposes; however, its role is limited because of noniodine-avid tumor that can be seen frequently in thyroid carcinoma because of genetic de-differentiation of the tumor cells. FDG-PET is an alternative in such patients for localizing locally persistent disease as well as distant metastasis. PET improves the diagnostic accuracy, aids in the development of optimal treatment strategies, and provides prognostic information. Dual imaging either with CT or MR imaging (PET/CT, PET/MR imaging) would increase the clinical impact of FDG-PET in patients with minimal cervical adenopathy and small pulmonary metastases.

REFERENCES

1. Parkin MD, Pisani P, Ferlay J. Global cancer statistics. Cancer J Clin 1999;49:33–64.
2. Hundahl SA, Fleming ID, Fremgen AM, et al. A National Cancer Data Base report on 53,856 cases of thyroid carcinoma treated in the US, '85–'95. Cancer 1998;83:2638–48.
3. Ron E, Kleinerman RA, Boice JD Jr, et al. A population based case-control study of thyroid cancer. J Natl Cancer Inst 1987;79:1–12.
4. Shore RE. Issues and epidemiologic evidence regarding radiation-induced thyroid cancer. Radiat Res 1992;131:98–111.
5. Fraker DL, Skarulis M, Livolsi V. Thyroid tumors. In: De-Vita VT, Hellman S, Rosenberg SA, editors. Cancer—principles and practice of oncology. 5th edition. Philadelphia: Lippincott-Raven; 1997. p. 1629–51.
6. Hundahl SA. Perspective: National Cancer Institute summary about estimated exposures and thyroid doses received from iodine-131 in fallout after Nevada atmospheric nuclear bomb tests. Cancer J Clin 1998;48:285–98.
7. Hamilton TE, van Belle G, LoGerfo JP. Thyroid neoplasia in Marshall islanders exposed to nuclear fallout. JAMA 1987;258:629–36.
8. Nikiforov Y, Gnepp DR. Pediatric thyroid cancer after the Chernobyl disaster. Cancer 1994;74:748–66.
9. Ron E, Lubin JH, Shore RE, et al. Thyroid cancer after exposure to external radiation: a pooled analysis of seven studies. Radiat Res 1995;141:259–77.
10. Schneider AB, Ron E. Pathogenesis. In: Braverman LE, Utiger RD, editors. Werner and Ingbars the thyroid: a fundamental and clinical text. 7th edition. Philadelphia: Lippincott-Raven; 1996. p. 902–6.
11. Francheschi S, Boyle P, Maisonneuve P, et al. The epidemiology of thyroid carcinoma. Crit Rev Oncog 1993;4:25–52.
12. Chung J-K, So Y, Lee JS, et al. Value of FDG-PET in papillary thyroid carcinoma with negative 131-I whole-body scan. J Nucl Med 1999;40:986–92.
13. Grunwald F, Menzel C, Bender H, et al. Comparison of F-18 FDG-PET with iodine-131 and Tc-99m-sestamibi scintigraphy in differentiated thyroid cancer. Thyroid 1997;7:327–35.
14. Dietlein M, Scheidhauer K, Voth E, et al. Fluorine-18-fluorodeoxyglucose positron emission tomography and iodine-131 whole-body scintigraphy in the follow-up of differentiated thyroid cancer. Eur J Nucl Med 1997;24:1342–8.

15. Grunwald F, Schomburg A, Bender H, et al. Fluorine-18 fluorodexyglucose positron emission tomography in the follow-up of differentiated thyroid cancer. Eur J Nucl Med 1996;23:312–9.

16. Anderson GS, Fish S, Nakhoda K, et al. Comparison of I-123 and I-131 600 for whole-body imaging after stimulation by recombinant human thyrotropin: a preliminary report. Clin Nucl Med 2003;28:93–6.

17. Urhan M, Dadparvar S, Mavi A, et al. I-123 As a diagnostic imaging agent in differentiated thyroid carcinoma: a comparison with i-131 post-treatment scanning and serum thyroglobulin measurement. Eur J Nucl Med Mol Imaging 2007;34(7):1012–7.

18. Dai G, Levy O, Carrasco N. Cloning and characterization of the thyroid iodide transporter. Nature 1996;379:458–60.

19. Casara D, Rubello D, Saladini G, et al. Clinical approach in patients with metastatic differentiated thyroid carcinoma and negative I-131 whole body scintigraphy: importance of Tc-99m MIBI scan combined with high resolution neck US. Tumori 1999;85:120–5.

20. Baudin E, Schulumberger M, Lumbroso J, et al. Octreotide scintigraphy in patients with differentiated thyroid carcinoma: contribution for patients with negative radioiodine scans. J Clin Endocrinol Metab 1996;81:2541–4.

21. Burman KD, Anderson JH, Wartofsky L, et al. Management of patients with thyroid carcinoma: application of Tl-201 scintigraphy and magnetic resonance imaging. J Nucl Med 1990;31:1958–64.

22. Dadparvar S, Chevres A, Thulchinsky M, et al. Clinical Utility of Tc-99m MIBI imaging in differentiated thyroid carcinoma: comparison with Tl-201 and I-131 Na scintigraphy and serum thyroglobulin quantitation. Eur J Nucl Med 1995;22:1330–8.

23. Warburg O. The metabolism of tumors. London: Constable; 1930.

24. Lowe VJ, Fletcher JW, Gobar L, et al. Prospective investigation of positron emission tomography in lung nodules. J Clin Oncol 1998;16(3):1075–84.

25. Hall N, Kloos RT. PET Imaging in differentiated thyroid cancer: where does it fit and how do we use it? Arq Bras Endocrinol Metabol 2007;51(5):793–805.

26. Coleman PM, Babb P, Damiecky P, et al. Cancer survival trends in England and Wales 1971–1995: deprivation and NHS region series SMPS no: 61. London: Stationary Office; 1999. p. 471–8.

27. Krishnamurthy S, Bedi DG, Caraway NP. Ultrasound-guided fine-needle aspiration of the thyroid bed. Cancer 2001;25:199–205.

28. Kang KW, Kim SK, Kang HS, et al. Prevalence and risk of cancer of focal thyroid incidentaloma identified by 18F-fluorodeoxyglucose positron emission tomography for metastasis evaluation and cancer screening in healthy subjects. J Clin Endocrinol Metab 2003;88:4100–4.

29. Kim TY, Kim WB, Ryu JS, et al. 18Ffluorodeoxyglucose uptake in thyroid from positron emission tomogram (PET) for evaluation in cancer patients: high prevalence of malignancy in thyroid PET incidentaloma. Laryngoscope 2005;115:1074–8.

30. Chen YK, Ding HJ, Chen KT, et al. Prevalence and risk of cancer of focal thyroid incidentaloma identified by 18F-fluorodeoxyglucose positron emission tomography for cancer screening in healthy subjects. Anticancer Res 2005;25:1421–6.

31. Choi JY, Lee KS, Kim HJ, et al. Focal thyroid lesions incidentally identified by integrated 18FFDG PET/CT: clinical significance and improved characterization. J Nucl Med 2006;47:609–15.

32. Adler LP, Bloom AD. Positron emission tomography of thyroid masses. Thyroid 1993;3:195–200.

33. Bloom AD, Adler LP, Shuck JM. Determination of malignancy of thyroid nodules with positron emission tomography. Surgery 1993;114:728–34.

34. Scott GC, Meier DA, Dickinson CZ. Cervical lymph node metastasis of thyroid papillary carcinoma imaged with fluorine-18-FDG, technetium-99m-pertechnetate and iodine-131-sodium iodide. J Nucl Med 1995;36:1843–5.

35. Cooper DS, Doherty GM, Haugen BR, et al. Management guidelines for patients with thyroid nodules and differentiated thyroid cancer. Thyroid 2006;16(2):109–41.

36. Geus-Oei LF, Pieters GF, Bonenkamp JJ, et al. 18F-FDG PET reduces unnecessary hemithyroidectomies for thyroid nodules with inconclusive cytologic results. J Nucl Med 2006;47:770–5.

37. Kim JM, Ryu JS, Kim TY, et al. 18F-luorodeoxyglucose positron emission tomography does not predict malignancy in thyroid nodules cytologically diagnosed as follicular neoplasm. J Clin Endocrinol Metab 2007;92(5):1630–4.

38. Kresnik E, Gallowitsch HJ, Mikosch P, et al. Fluorine-18-fluorodeoxyglucose positron emission tomography in the preoperative assessment of thyroid nodules in an endemic goiter area. Surgery 2003;133:294–9.

39. Joensuu H, Ahonen A. Imaging of metastases of thyroid carcinoma with fluorine-18 fluorodeoxyglucose. J Nucl Med 1987;28:910–4.

40. Feine U, Lietzenmayer R, Hanke JP, et al. Fluorine-18-FDG and iodine-131-iodide uptake in thyroid cancer. J Nucl Med 1996;37:1468–72.

41. Grunwald F, Kalicke T, Feine U, et al. Fluorine-18 fluorodeoxyglucose positron emission tomography in thyroid cancer: results of a multicentre study. Eur J Nucl Med 1999;26:1547–52.

42. Wang WP, Macapinlac H, Larson SM, et al. F-18 -2-fluoro-2-deoxy-D-glucose positron emission tomography localizes residual thyroid cancer in patients with negative diagnostic I-131 whole body scans and elevated serum thyroglobulin levels. J Clin Endocrinol Metab 1999;84:2291–302.

43. Frilling A, Tecklenborg K, Görges R, et al. Preoperative diagnostic value of [(18)F] fluorodeoxyglucose positron emission tomography in patients with radio-iodine-negative recurrent well-differentiated thyroid carcinoma. Ann Surg 2001;234(6):804–11.

44. Shiga T, Tsukamoto E, Nakada K, et al. Comparison of 18-F-FDG, 131-I-Na and 201-Tl in diagnosis of recurrent or metastatic thyroid carcinoma. J Nucl Med 2001;42:414–9.

45. Yeo JS, Chung JK, So Y, et al. F-18-fluoro-deoxy-glucose positron emission tomography as a presurgical evaluation modality for I-131 negative thyroid carcinoma patients with local recurrence in cervical lymph nodes. Head Neck 2001;23:94–103.

46. Schluter B, Bohuslavizki KH, Beyer W, et al. Impact of FDG-PET on patients with differentiated thyroid cancer who present with elevated thyroglobulin and negative 131I scan. J Nucl Med 2001;42:71–6.

47. Helal BO, Merlet P, Toubert ME, et al. Clinical impact of (18)F-FDG-PET in thyroid carcinoma patients with elevated thyroglobulin levels and negative (131)I scanning results after therapy. J Nucl Med 2001; 42:1464–9.

48. Plotkin M, Hautzel H, Krause BJ, et al. Implication of 2-(18)fluor-2-deoxyglucose positron emission tomography in the follow-up of Hurtle cell thyroid cancer. Thyroid 2002;12:155–61.

49. Sarlis NJ, Gourgiotis I, Guthrie LC, et al. In-111 DTPA- octreotide scintigraphy for disease detection in metastatic thyroid cancer: comparison with F-18 FDG positron emission tomography and extensive conventional radiographic imaging. Clin Nucl Med 2003;28:208–17.

50. Chen YK, Liu FY, Yen RF, et al. Compare FDG-PET and Tc-99m tetrafosmin SPECT to detect metastatic thyroid carcinoma. Acad Radiol 2003;10:835–9.

51. Hung MC, Wu HS, Kao CH, et al. F-18-fluoro-deoxyglucose positron emission tomography in detecting metastatic papillary thyroid carcinoma with elevated human serum thyroglobulin levels but negative I-131 whole-body scan. Endocr Res 2003; 29:169–75.

52. Gabriel M, Froehlich F, Decristoforo C, et al. 99mTc-EDDA/HYNIC-TOC and (18)F-FDG in thyroid cancer patients with negative (131)I whole-body scans. Eur J Nucl Med Mol Imaging 2004;31:330–41.

53. Nahas Z, Goldenberg D, Fakhry C, et al. The role of positron emission tomography/computed tomography in the management of recurrent papillary thyroid carcinoma. Laryngoscope 2005;115:237–43.

54. Pryma DA, Schoder H, Gonen M, et al. Diagnostic accuracy and prognostic value of 18F-FDG PET in Hurtle cell thyroid cancer. J Nucl Med 2006;47(8):1260–6.

55. Shammas A, Degirmenci B, Mountz JM, et al. 18F-FDG PET/CT in patients with suspected recurrent or metastatic well-differentiated thyroid cancer. J Nucl Med 2007;48(2):221–6.

56. Salvatore B, Paone G, Klain M, et al. Fluorodeoxyglucose positron emission tomography/computed tomography in patients with differentiated thyroid cancer and elevated thyroglobulin after total thyroidectomy and 131-I ablation. Q J Nucl Med Mol Imaging 2007;51:1–7.

57. Iagaru A, Kalinyak JE, McDougall IR. F-18 FDG PET/CT in the management of thyroid cancer. Clin Nucl Med 2007;32:690–5.

58. Zoller M, Kohlfuerst S, Igerc I, et al. Combined PET/CT in the follow-up of differentiated thyroid carcinoma: what is the impact of each modality? Eur J Nucl Med Mol Imaging 2007;34:487–95.

59. Azadian A, Rosen IB, Walfish PG, et al. Management consideration in Hurtle cell carcinoma. Surgery 1995;118:711–4.

60. Shaha AR, Ferlito A, Rinaldo A. Distant metastases from thyroid and parathyroid cancer. ORL J Otorhinolaryngol Relat Spec 2001;63:243–9.

61. Yen TC, Lin HD, Lee CH, et al. The role of Technetium-99m sestamibi whole-body scans in diagnosing metastatic Hurtle cell carcinoma of the thyroid gland after total thyroidectomy: a comparison with iodine-131 and thallium-201whole-body scans. Eur J Nucl Med 1994;21:980–3.

62. Jadvar H, Fishman AJ. Evaluation of rare tumors with (F-18)fluorodeoxyglucose positron emission tomography. Clin Positron Imaging 1999;2:153–8.

63. McDougall IR, Jadvar H, Segall G. PET scan in patients with suspected recurrent thyroid cancer. Presented at thyroid one. Thyroid Cancer Pathogenesis, Diagnosis including PET, and treatment. International Symposium. Linz, Austria, October 7–10, 1998. Thyroid 1998;8:1222, Abstract.

64. Zimmer LA, McCook B, Meltzer C, et al. Combined positron emission tomography/computed tomography imaging of recurrent thyroid cancer. Otolaryngol Head Neck Surg 2003;128:178–84.

65. Wang W, Larson SM, Fazzari M, et al. Prognostic value of 18-F-Fluorodeoxyglucose positron emission tomographic scanning in patients with thyroid cancer. J Clin Endocrinol Metab 2000;85:1107–13.

66. Schonberger J, Ruschhoff J, Grimm D, et al. Glucose transporter-1 gene expression is related to thyroid neoplasm with an unfavorable prognosis: an immunohistochemical study. Thyroid 2002;12: 747–54.

67. Giammarile F, Hafdi Z, Bournaud C, et al. Is 18F -2-fluoro-2-deoxy-D-glucose (FDG) scintigraphy with non-dedicated positron emission tomography useful in the diagnostic management of suspected metastatic thyroid carcinoma in patients with no detectable radioiodine uptake? Eur J Endocrinol 2003;149:293–300.

68. Lowe VJ, Mullan BP, Hay ID, et al. 18F-FDG PET of patients with Hurtle-cell carcinoma. J Nucl Med 2003;44:1402–6.

69. Schluter B, Grimm-Riepe C, Beyer W, et al. Histological verification of positive fluorine-18 fluorodeoxyglucose findings in patients with differentiated thyroid cancer. Langenbecks Arch Surg 1998;383: 187–9, 692.

70. Muros MA, Llamas-Elvira JM, Ramirez-Navarro A, et al. Utility of fluorine-18-fluorodeoxyglucose positron emission tomography in differentiated thyroid carcinoma with negative radioiodine scans and elevated serum thyroglobulin levels. Am J Surg 2000;179:457–61.

71. Pacini F, Schlumberger M, Dralle H, et al. European Consensus for the management of patients with differentiated thyroid carcinoma of the follicular epithelium. Eur J endocrinol 2006;154:787–803.

72. Haraguchi K, Rani CS, Field JB. Effects of thyrotropin, carbachol, and protein kinase-C stimulators on glucose transport and glucose oxidation by primary cultures of dog thyroid cells. Endocrinology 1988; 123:1288–95.

73. Filetti S, Damante G, Foti D. Thyrotropin stimulates glucose transport in cultured rat thyroid cells. Endocrinology 1987;120:2576–81.

74. Hosaka Y, Tawata M, Kurlhara A, et al. The regulation of two distinct glucose transporter (GLUT1 and GLUT4) gene expression in cultured rat thyroid cells by thyrotropin. Endocrinology 1992;131: 159–65.

75. Sisson JC, Ackermann RJ, Meyer MA, et al. Uptake of 18-fluoro-2-deoxy-D-glucose by thyroid cancer. Implications for diagnosis and therapy. J Clin Endocrinol Metab 1993;77:1090–4.

76. Eustatia-Rytten CF, Smit JW, Romijn JA, et al. Diagnostic value of serum thyroglobulin measurements in the follow-up of differentiated thyroid carcinoma, a structured meta-analysis. Clin Endocrinol (Oxf) 2004;61:61–74.

77. van Tol KM, Jager PL, Piers DA, et al. Better yield of (18)fluo-fluorodeoxyglucose-positron emission tomography in patients with metastatic differentiated thyroid carcinoma during thyrotropin stimulation. Thyroid 2002;715(12):381–7.

78. Chin BB, Patel P, Cohade C, et al. Recombinant human thyrotropin stimulation of fluoro-D-glucose positron emission tomography uptake in well-differentiated thyroid carcinoma. J Clin Endocrinol Metab 2004;89:91–5.

79. Moog F, Linke R, Manthey N, et al. Influence of thyroid-stimulating hormone levels on uptake of FDG in recurrent and metastatic differentiated thyroid carcinoma. J Nucl Med 2000;41:1989–95.

80. Petrich T, Borner AR, Weckesser E, et al. Follow-up of thyroid cancer patients using rhTSH: preliminary results. Nuklearmedizin 2001;40:7–14.

81. Lambrecht RM, Woodhouse N, Phillips R, et al. Investigational study of iodine-124 with a positron camera. Am J Physiol Imaging 1988;3:197–200.

82. Pentlow KS, Graham MC, Lambrecht RM, et al. Quantative imaging of iodine-124 with PET. J Nucl Med 1996;37:1557–62.

83. Frey P, Townsend D, Flattet A, et al. Tomographic imaging of the human thyroid using 124I. J Clin Endocrinol Metab 1986;63:918–27.

84. Schmidt D, Herzog H, Langen K-J, et al. Glucose metabolism in thyroid cancer metastases. A pilot study using 18 fluoro-2-deoxy-D-glucose and positron emission tomography. Exp Clin Endocrinol 1994;102:51–4.

85. Pacini F, Molinaro E, Castagna MG, et al. Recombinant human thyrotropin-stimulated serum thyroglobulin combined with neck ultrasonography has the highest sensitivity in monitoring differentiated thyroid carcinoma. J Clin Endocrinol Metab 2003;88:3668–73.

86. Palmedo H, Bucerius J, Joe A, et al. Integrated PET/CT in differentiated thyroid cancer: diagnostic accuracy and impact on patient management. J Nucl Med 2006;47:616–24.

87. Halpern BS, Yeom K, Fueger BJ, et al. Evaluation of suspected local recurrence in head and neck cancer: a comparison between PET and PET/CT for biopsy proven lesions. Eur J Radiol 2007;62:199–204.

88. Ilgan S, Karacalıoglu AO, Pabuscu Y, et al. Iodine-131 treatment and high resolution CT: results in patients with lung metastases from differentiated thyroid carcinoma. Eur J Nucl Med Mol Imaging 2004;31:825–30.

89. Bar-Shalom R, Yefremov N, Guralnik L, et al. Clinical performance of PET/CT in evaluation of cancer: additional value for diagnostic imaging and patient management. J Nucl Med 2003;44:1200–9.

90. Nakamoto Y, Cohade C, Tatsumi M, et al. CT appearance of bone metastases detected with FDG-PET as part of the same PET/CT examination. Radiology 2005;237:627–34.

91. Schirrmeister H, Guhlman A, Elsner K, et al. Sensitivity in detecting osseous lesions depends on anatomic localization: planar bone scintigraphy versus 18-F PET. J Nucl Med 1990;40:1623–9.

The Evolving Role of Positron Emission Tomography in Patients with Medullary Thyroid Carcinoma

Muammer Urhan, MD[a],*, Abass Alavi, MD, PhD[b],
Cristina Nanni, MD[c]

KEYWORDS

- Positron emission tomography • Medullary thyroid cancer
- FDG • F-DOPA

Medullary thyroid carcinoma (MTC) is a rare tumor of calcitonin-secreting parafollicular C-cells, and it has a poor prognosis compared with follicular cell–derived tumors. It comprises 3.5% to 7% of all thyroid malignancies but accounts for up to 17% of all cancer deaths. Total thyroidectomy is the treatment of choice, and the prognosis is closely related to the stage of the disease at initial diagnosis. After thyroidectomy, the sequential measurement of serum calcitonin has been highly sensitive and specific for monitoring effects of treatment and detecting active disease. It is important to localize the sites of disease precisely for subsequent surgical intervention; however, measurement of calcitonin levels in the blood provides no information about the location of active disease. Positron emission tomography (PET) with ^{18}F-fluorodeoxyglucose (FDG) has been useful in localizing metastatic spread to the cervical and mediastinal lymph nodes and revealing distant metastatic sites.

FDG-PET imaging leads to a change in the management of patients with this disease by excluding local or distant metastases for which surgery is the only possible cure. Some authors have suggested a comparison between serum calcitonin concentrations and PET imaging results. FDG-PET scan has a reported sensitivity as high as 78%. Anatomic and metabolic information provided by dedicated hybrid imaging systems, such as PET/CT or PET/MR imaging, may improve the sensitivity of the procedure, especially in the head and neck region, for fine needle aspiration and lymph node dissection. Other PET tracers may be useful for detecting recurrent of metastatic disease in patients with MCT, such as carbon-11 (C-11) hydroxyltriptophan, C-11 3,4-dihydroxy-L-phenylalanin (DOPA), and 18-F DOPA. Preliminary data obtained from 18-F-DOPA studies are promising and seem more sensitive than ^{18}F-FDG PET in localizing persistent disease in patients who have MTC.

MTC is a rare tumor that originates from calcitonin-producing parafollicular C-cells. The disease is inherited as an autosomal dominant trait associated with other endocrine neoplasms in approximately 20% of patients, but the remaining 80% of individuals who have MTC are afflicted by a sporadic, nonfamilial form of the disease.[1] Histology in MTC is characterized by sheets of

[a] Department of Nuclear Medicine, GATA Haydarpasa Training Hospital, Selimiye Mah Tibbiye Cad 34668 Uskudar, Istanbul, Turkey

[b] Division of Nuclear Medicine, Department of Radiology, Hospital of the University of Pennsylvania, 3400 Spruce Street, 110 Donner Building, Philadelphia, PA 19104, USA

[c] UO Medicina Nucleare, Azienda Ospedaliero-Universitaria di Bologna Policlinico S.Orsola-Malpighi, Bologna, Italy

* Corresponding author. Division of Nuclear Medicine, GATA Haydarpasa Training Hospital, Selimiye Mah Tibbiye Cad 34668 Uskadar, Istanbul, Turkey.
E-mail address: urhanm@gmail.com (M. Urhan).

PET Clin 2 (2008) 305–311
doi:10.1016/j.cpet.2008.04.006

cells with large nuclei, deposition of amyloid, and extensive fibrosis. A wide range of morphologic patterns, such as pseudo-papillary, spindle cell, trabecular, and tubular variants, are noted on histologic examination. The parafollicular C-cells in the neuroendocrine tumors are characterized by amine precursor uptake and decarboxylation and are capable of producing, storing, and releasing various neuropeptides, including calcitonin, somatostatin, adrenocorticotropic hormone, gastrin-releasing peptide, and carcinoembryonic antigen.[2] The prognosis of MTC is relatively poor compared with the other forms of well-differentiated thyroid carcinoma. MTC comprises 3.5% to 7% of all thyroid malignancies but accounts for approximately 17% of all thyroid cancer deaths.[3,4] The sporadic and inherited forms usually have the same prognosis, which is more favorable in young patients (< 40 years); however, multiple endocrine neoplasia type 2B has a relatively poorer outcome.[5] The only potentially curative treatment for MTC is surgery, and total thyroidectomy is recommended for preoperatively diagnosed medullary carcinoma. The prognosis is good when the tumor is totally confined to the thyroid gland and detected at an early stage. Some surgeons recommend prophylactic central lymph node dissection and even proceed to a modified neck dissection because local invasion to cervical and mediastinal lymph nodes already has been detected in approximately 35% of the patients at the time of initial diagnosis. The overall 10-year survival rate is approximately 90% if the tumor is confined to the thyroid and 70% and 20% in cases of lymphatic spread and distant metastasis, respectively.[6,7]

DETECTION OF RECURRENT MEDULLARY THYROID CARCINOMA

Selective venous sampling and monitoring of serum calcitonin levels are used to determine the side of the neck to be dissected by the surgeon.[8–11] This procedure, however, is invasive and requires specialized skills.

Cervical ultrasound is usually the first-line anatomic imaging method because the procedure is easy to perform and may detect local invasion of surrounding structures by MTC. With sonography, the detection rate of residual or metastatic lesions in the neck varies from 78% to 96%.[12,13] Tomographic imaging modalities, such as CT and MR imaging, also have proven to be sensitive procedures for imaging the thyroid bed and cervical lymph nodes, especially for lesions approximately 1 cm in size. The sensitivities of CT and MR imaging have been found to be 38% to 70% and 44%

to 74%, respectively. Detection of residual tumor and lymph node metastasis in the cervical and mediastinal areas is difficult after surgery. After thyroidectomy, a reliable differentiation between the postoperative changes and recurrent tumor in the thyroid bed poses a challenge for anatomic imaging modalities alone.[14–17] Cervical dissection is successful only in the absence of distant metastases, which may not be seen by anatomic imaging alone.

In contrast, functional imaging by nuclear medicine modalities is not affected by postoperative changes and permits whole-body scanning for metastases. The sensitivity of nuclear imaging with somatostatin receptor compounds,[18–22] technetium 99m Tc–labeled pentavalent dimercaptosuccinic acid (^{Tc}99m DMSA-V),[23,24] metaiodobenzylguanidine (MIBG) labeled with either I-131 or I-123, metoxyisobuthyl-isonitril (^{Tc}99m MIBI), and thalium 201 Tl chloride (^{Tl}201 chloride)[25–29] has varied from 25% to 95%. New approaches and radiotracers, such as radiolabeled anti- carcinoembryonic antigen antibodies and gastrin receptor scintigraphy, have been used in patients who have MTC, but they have been noted to be of limited value in this malignancy.[30–35]

PET is a functional imaging modality that has been increasingly used in clinical oncology.[36] ^{18}F-FDG, a glucose analog, has been used successfully to detect malignant cells because of their increased glucose metabolism influenced by the grade of differentiation. It is transported across the cell membrane by glucose transporters (GLUT 1) and phosphorylated to FDG-6-P by hexokinase. FDG-6-P can neither enter the upper glycolytic pathways nor diffuse back to the extracellular space, and it is inside the cell for an extended period of time.

FDG-PET can be used as a noninvasive modality for preoperative staging and postoperative follow-up, especially in patients who have MTC with high or elevated serum calcitonin levels (**Figs. 1** and **2**). Studies have investigated the potential role of FDG-PET in patients who have MTC and have compared the results with those of conventional nuclear medicine and anatomic imaging techniques.[37–40] A study by de Groot and colleagues[41] reported that FDG-PET was superior to conventional nuclear imaging, including pentavalent technetium 99m Tc DMSA and indium 111 In–labeled octreotide and bone scintigraphy in detecting MTC lesions. They postulated that FDG-PET can replace conventional nuclear medicine procedures as the method of choice because of its superior performance.

In some studies, FDG-PET has been compared with anatomic imaging modalities, especially in

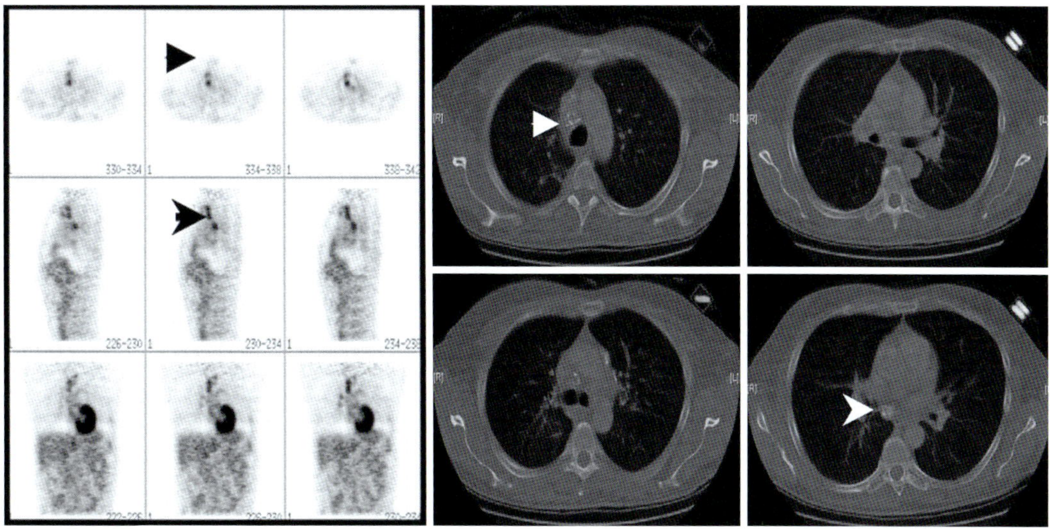

Fig. 1. A 53-year-old man with mediastinal FDG uptake consistent with metastasis, which was confirmed by CT.

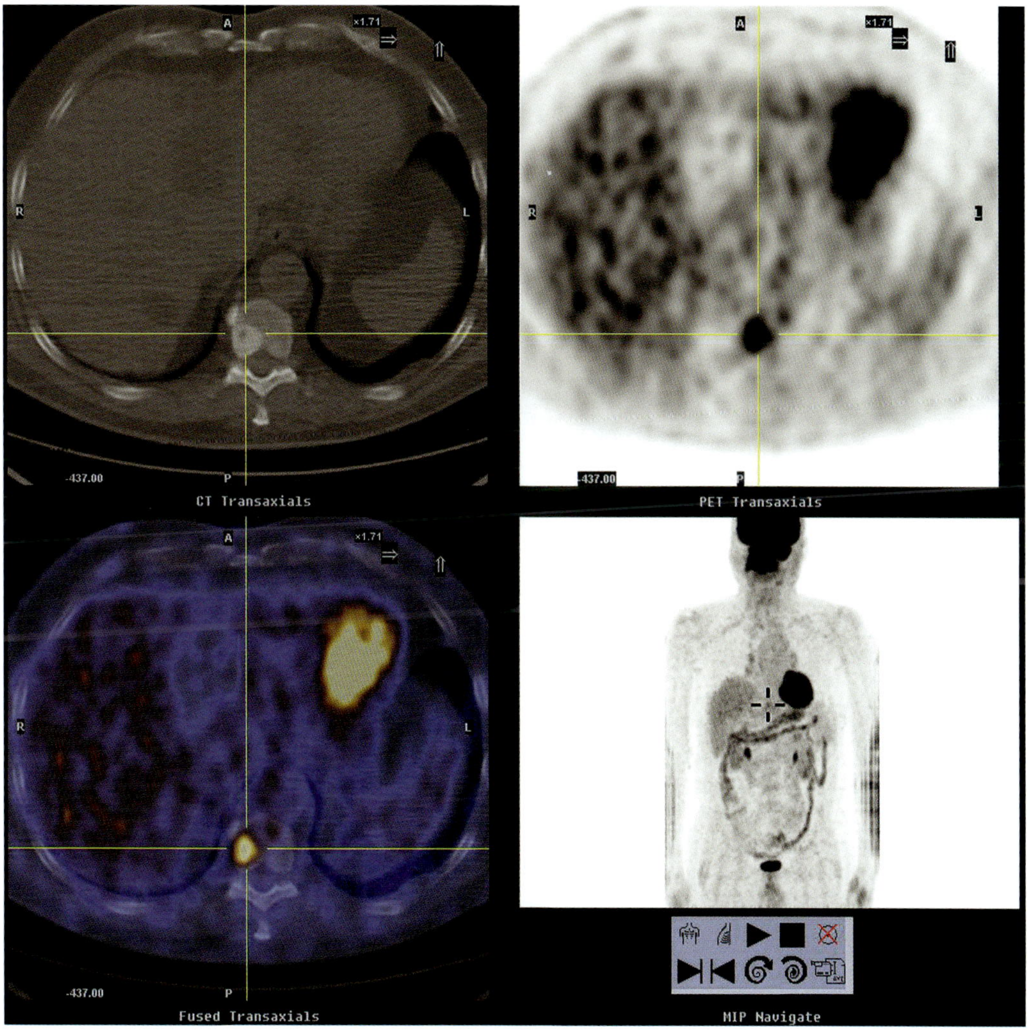

Fig. 2. Metastatic MTC detected by FDG-PET/CT in the spine. The disease was visualized on both modalities.

identifying lymph node metastasis. Sensitivities as high as 78% have been reported.[42] Szakall and colleagues[43] reported that FDG-PET detected more cervical, supraclavicular, and mediastinal lesions than did structural imaging methods. It also been has reported that FDG-PET failed to localize small metastatic lesions, especially those smaller than 1 cm, in organs such as the liver and the lung. This finding suggests that anatomic and functional imaging modalities have advantages and disadvantages in assessing this malignancy. In organs such as the lungs, lesions can be detected readily by CT and MR imaging because of their superior spatial resolution. The specificity of these techniques is low in assessing lymph nodes and after surgical and other interventions.[44]

FDG-PET whole-body scanning has the advantage of not only detecting disease activity in the operative site but also evaluating for distant organ metastasis. Structural imaging with ultrasound, CT, and MR imaging is of limited value in certain settings with this cancer. FDG-PET can complement anatomic imaging by providing metabolic information and contribute significantly to the identification of recurrent or metastatic MTC. Anatomic and metabolic information can be provided by combined PET/CT imaging in a single session, and as a result the specificity of the structural imaging alone is improved. PET/CT and PET/MR imaging are useful in the localization of active disease in most locations. The information provided by coregistering the morphologic and functional imaging techniques enables a precise fine needle biopsy preoperatively and allows a surgeon to plan an effective approach when the anatomy of the neck has been altered by previous surgical intervention.[45–47]

Despite the data in the literature indicating that FDG-PET can be used to detect recurrent MTC, some authors postulate that it may be less useful in investigating certain neuroendocrine tumors.[48] MTC illustrates several characteristics of neuroendocrine tumors,[2] which may explain the false-negative FDG-PET results in patients who have MTC. It was previously reported that there is an inverse correlation between the degree of dedifferentiation and the level of glucose metabolism. By now it is well established that many well-differentiated tumor of some organs are depicted with poor sensitivity by FDG-PET because of normal or low glucose metabolism in these cancers.[49,50] Musholt and colleagues[51,52] reported that the expression of glucose transporter proteins GLUT 1-5 was not increased in MTC; however, FDG-PET imaging could be used to localize cervicomediastinal invasion.

For a long time it has been known that neuroendocrine tumors are capable of metabolizing amino acids to biogenic amines by a decarboxylation process and storing them in vesicles.[53,54] Promising results have been reported in gastrointestinal neuroendocrine tumors using PET tracers, such as C-11 hydroxyltriptophan, C-11 DOPA, and F-18 DOPA (**Fig. 3**).[53,55–57] Among

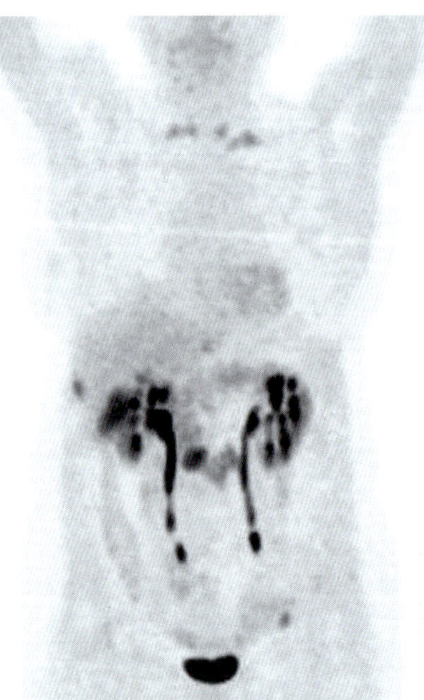
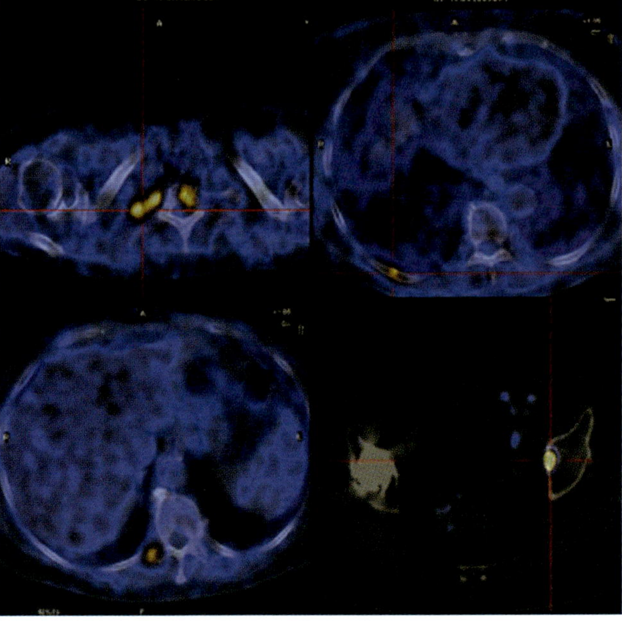

Fig. 3. MTC with progressive increase in serum tumor markers with negative results on conventional imaging techniques and positive results on F-DOPA-PET with multiple metastatic bone marrow lesions.

these preparations, F-18 DOPA has been used successfully to examine patients with metastasizing ileal carcinoid because of its relatively long half-life and availability for routine clinical use.[58] A study by Hoegerle and colleagues[59] reported that F-18 DOPA-PET imaging has a higher sensitivity than FDG-PET (63% versus 44%) and complements the information provided by anatomic imaging techniques in patients with primary or recurrent MTC.

In approximately one-half of the cases, F-18 DOPA-PET was able to localize additional lesions or optimally characterize the lesions seen on anatomic imaging as benign or suspicious for malignancy. F-18 DOPA-PET also has failed to reveal liver metastases in some patients; tumor dedifferentiation has been postulated as a possible explanation for this observation.

Beuthien-Baumann and colleagues[60] reported the use of FDG, F-18 DOPA, and 3-O-methyl -6-18F-fluoro-DOPA (F-18 OMFD) in 15 patients with elevated calcitonin levels to assess the possible uptake mechanisms in MTC cells. F-18 OMFD has been used for brain tumor imaging. This agent is not taken up by any organ systems in the thorax or abdomen and is excreted by the kidneys rapidly, which results in high contrast and relatively low radiation exposure to the body.[61]

In the study by Beuthien-Baumann and colleagues, a large discrepancy was noted with regard to the sites of disease with these three compounds. FDG accumulates in the inflammatory cells in nonmalignant tissues, which show no uptake of amino acid analogs. The degree of differentiation in MTC cells is another explanation for differing tracer uptake by tumor cells. Similar to other forms of follicular cell–derived thyroid carcinoma, it has been assumed that more FDG is taken up in poorly differentiated tumors, whereas F-18 DOPA–positive lesions express a higher degree of differentiation.[39,62] On the other hand, they reported that F-18 OMFD had no diagnostic value in ten patients who had MTC. The size of the population examined makes it difficult to make a definite conclusion about the role of these compounds in MTC.[60]

Gourgiotis and colleagues[63] reported a positive result in a biopsy-proven MTC recurrence in a patient with multiple endocrine neoplasia type 2A by using 6-F-18 fluorodopamine, a novel PET tracer that has been useful in investigating chromaffin tumors such as pheochromocytomas. The uptake mechanism depends on the assumption that up to 35% of MTCs concentrate MIBG and the norepinephrine transporter system can take up MIBG and 6-F-18 fluorodopamine.[64]

FOLLOW-UP OF RECURRENT MEDULLARY THYROID CARCINOMA

Approximately 6 weeks after surgery, calcitonin levels should be checked to determine the degree of success of the intervention. A decrease in serum concentration or a serum concentration in the normal range suggests favorable outcome, whereas high levels of tumor markers, such as calcitonin or carcinoembryonic antigen, strongly suggest persistent MTC. Calcitonin is a highly sensitive and specific marker for persistent tumor but gives no localization information for further intervention. Molecular imaging techniques described in this communication may play a major role in the follow-up of these patients.

SUMMARY

Surgery is the only curative option available to individuals who have MTC, and the precise localization of recurrent or metastatic lesions is important in their management. So far no single imaging modality has been successful in the initial staging or identification of persistent disease. Various structural and functional modalities have been used for this purpose. A combination of anatomic and functional imaging procedures is likely to provide the most optimal information for clinical assessment of these patients. In combination with anatomic imaging, FDG-PET imaging has been the most preferred procedure for localizing recurrent or metastatic MTC in patients with elevated serum calcitonin levels. Some promising results have been observed using the new tracers, such as F-18 DOPA, however.

REFERENCES

1. Bustros AC, Baylin SB. Medullary carcinoma of thyroid. In: Braverman LE, Utiger RD, editors. Werner and Ingbar's the thyroid. New York: JB Lippincott Company; 1991. p. 1167.
2. Modigliani E, Cohen R, Campos JM, et al. Prognostic factors for survival and for biochemical cure in medullary thyroid carcinoma: results in 899 patients. The GETC Study Group. Group d'etude des tumeurs a calcitonine. Clin Endocrin (Oxf) 1998;48:265–73.
3. Correa P, Chen VW. Endocrine gland cancer. Cancer 1995;75:338–52.
4. Marsh DJ, Learoyd DL, Robinson BG. Medullary thyroid carcinoma: recent advances and management update. Thyroid 1995;5:407–24.
5. O'Riordain DS, O'Brien T, Weaver AL, et al. Medullary thyroid carcinoma in multiple endocrine neoplasia types 2A and 2B. Surgery 1994;116:1017–23.
6. Saad MF, Ordonez NG, Rashid RK, et al. Medullary carcinoma of the thyroid: a study of the clinical

and prognostic factors in 161 patients. Medicine 1984;63:319–42.

7. Lairmore TC, Wells SA Jr. Medullary carcinoma of the thyroid: current diagnosis and management. Semin Surg Oncol 1991;7:92–9.

8. Grauer A, Raue F, Gagel R. Changing concepts in the management of hereditary and sporadic medullary carcinoma. Endocrinol Metab Clin North Am 1990;19:613–35.

9. Abdelmoumene N, Schlumberger M, Gardet P, et al. Selective venous sampling catheterisation for localisation of persisting medullary thyroid carcinoma. Br J Cancer 1994;69:1141–4.

10. Raue F, Winter J, Frank-Raue K, et al. Diagnostic procedure before reoperation in patients with medullary thyroid carcinoma. Horm Metab Res Suppl 1989;21:31–4.

11. Frank-Raue K, Raue F, Buhr HJ, et al. Localization of occult persisting medullary thyroid carcinoma before microsurgical reoperation: high sensitivity of selective venous catheterization. Thyroid 1992;2:113–7.

12. Norton JA, Doppman JL, Brennan MF. Localization and resection of clinically inapparent medullary carcinoma of the thyroid. Surgery 1980;87:616–22.

13. Simeone JF, Daniels GH, Hall DA, et al. Sonography in the follow-up of 100 patients with thyroid carcinoma. AJR Am J Roentgenol 1987;148:45–9.

14. Auffermann W, Clark OH, Thurnber S, et al. Recurrent thyroid carcinoma: characteristics on MR images. Radiology 1988;168:753–7.

15. Crow JP, Azar-Kia B, Prinz RA. Recurrent occult medullary thyroid carcinoma detected by MR imaging. AJR Am J Roentgenol 1989;152:1255–6.

16. Wang Q, Takashima S, Fukuda H, et al. Detection of medullary thyroid carcinoma and regional lymph node metastases by magnetic resonance imaging. Arch Otolaryngol Head Neck Surg 1999;125:842–8.

17. Stomper PL. Cancer imaging manual. Philadelphia: Lippincott; 1993. p. 51–60.

18. Dörr U, Würstlin S, Frank-Raue K, et al. Somatostatin receptor scintigraphy and magnetic resonance imaging in recurrent medullary thyroid carcinoma: a comparative study. Horm Metab Res Suppl 1993;27:48–55.

19. Baudin E, Lumbroso J, Schlumberger M, et al. Comparison of octreotide scintigraphy and conventional imaging in medullary thyroid carcinoma. J Nucl Med 1996;37:912–6.

20. Behr TM, Gotthardt M, Barth A, et al. Imaging tumors with peptide-based radioligands. Q J Nucl Med 2001;45:189–200.

21. Krausz Y, Rosler A, Guttmann H, et al. Somatostatin receptor scintigraphy for early detection of regional and distant metastases of medullary carcinoma of the thyroid. Clin Nucl Med 1999;24:256–60.

22. Berna L, Chico A, Matias-Guiu X, et al. Use of somatostatin analogue scintigraphy in the localization of recurrent medullary thyroid carcinoma. Eur J Nucl Med 1998;25:1482–8.

23. Arslan N, Ilgan S, Yuksel D, et al. Comparison of In-111 octreotide and Tc-99m (V) DMSA scintigraphy in the detection of medullary thyroid tumor foci in patients with elevated levels of tumor markers after surgery. Clin Nucl Med 2001;26:683–8.

24. Berna L, Cabezas R, Mora J, et al. 111In-octreotide and 99mTc(V)-dimercaptosuccinic acid studies in the imaging of recurrent medullary thyroid carcinoma. J Endocrinol 1995;144:339–45.

25. Limouris GS, Giannakopoulos V, Stavraka A, et al. Comparison of In-111 pentetreotide, Tc-99m (V)-DMSA and I-123 MIBG scintimaging in neural crest tumors. Anticancer Res 1997;17:1589–92.

26. Thomas CC, Cowan RJ, Albertson DA, et al. Detection of medullary carcinoma of the thyroid with I-131 MIBG. Clin Nucl Med 1994;19:1066–8.

27. Troncone L, Rufini V, Montemaggi P, et al. The diagnostic and therapeutic utility of radioiodinated meta-iodobenzylguanidine (MIBG): 5 years of experience. Eur J Nucl Med 1990;16:325–35.

28. Learoyd DL, Roach PJ, Briggs GM, et al. Technetium-99-sestamibi scanning in recurrent medullary thyroid carcinoma. J Nucl Med 1997;38:227–30.

29. Ugur Ö, Kostakoglu L, Güler N, et al. Comparison of 99mTc(V)-DMSA, 201Tl and 99mTc-MIBI imaging in the follow-up of patients with medullary carcinoma of the thyroid. Eur J Nucl Med 1996;23:1367–71.

30. Hoefnagel CA, Delprat CC, Zanin D, et al. New radionuclide tracers for the diagnosis and therapy of the medullary thyroid carcinoma. Clin Nucl Med 1988;13:159–65.

31. Manil L, Boudet F, Motte P, et al. Positive anticalcitonin immunoscintigraphy in patients with medullary thyroid carcinoma. Cancer Res 1989;49:5480–5.

32. Reiners C, Eilles C, Spiegel W, et al. Immunoscintigraphy in medullary thyroid cancer using an 123I- or 111In-labelled monoclonal anti-CEA antibody fragment. Nuklearmedizin 1986;25:227–31.

33. Peltier P, Curtet C, Chatal J-F, et al. Radioimmunodetection of medullary thyroid cancer using a bispecific anti-CEA/anti-indium-DTPA antibody and an indium-111-labeled DTPA dimer. J Nucl Med 1993;34:1267–73.

34. Behr TM, Jenner N, Radetzky S, et al. Targeting of cholecystokinin-B/gastrin receptors in vivo: preclinical and initial clinical evaluation of the diagnosis and therapeutic potential of radiolabelled gastrin. Eur J Nucl Med 1998;25:424–30.

35. Behr TM, Jenner J, Behe M, et al. Radiolabelled peptides for targeting cholecystokinin-B/gastrin receptor-expressing tumors. J Nucl Med 1999;40:1029–40.

36. Strauss LG, Conti PS. The application of PET in clinical oncology. J Nucl Med 1991;32:623–48.
37. Gasparoni P, Rubello D, Ferlin G. Potential role of fluorine-18-deoxyglucose (FDG) positron emission tomography (PET) in the staging of primitive and recurrent medullary thyroid carcinoma. J Endocrinol Invest 1997;20:527–30.
38. Diehl M, Risse JH, Brandt-Mainz K, et al. Fluorine-18 fluorodeoxyglucose positron emission tomography in medullary thyroid cancer: result of a multicenter study. Eur J Nucl Med 2001;28:1671–6.
39. Grünwald F, Kälicke T, Feine U, et al. Fluorine-18 fluorodeoxyglucose positron emission tomography in thyroid cancer: results of a multicenter study. Eur J Nucl Med 1999;26:1547–52.
40. Rufini V, Salvatori M, Garganese MC, et al. Role of nuclear medicine in the diagnosis and therapy of medullary thyroid carcinoma. Rays 2000;25:273–82.
41. de Groot JW, Links TP, Jager PL, et al. Impact of F-18 fluoro-2-deoxy-D-glucose positron emission tomography (FDG-PET) in patients with biochemical evidence of recurrent or residual medullary thyroid cancer. Ann Surg Oncol 2004;11(8):786–94.
42. Brandt-Mainz K, Muller SP, Gorges R, et al. The value of F-18 FDG PET in patients with medullary thyroid cancer. Eur J Nucl Med 2000;27:490–6.
43. Szakall S Jr, Esik O, Balzik G, et al. F-18 FDG-PET detection of lymph node metastases in medullary thyroid carcinoma. J Nucl Med 2002;43(1):66–71.
44. Crippa F, Alessi A, Gerali A, et al. FDG-PET in thyroid cancer. Tumori 2003;89:540–3.
45. Conti PS, Lilien DL, Hawley K, et al. PET and [18F]-FDG in oncology: a clinical update. Nucl Med Biol 1996;23:717–35.
46. Bockish A, Brandt-Mainz K, Görges R, et al. Diagnosis in medullary thyroid cancer with F-18 FDG-PET and improvent using a combined PET/CT scanner. Acta Med Austriaca 2003;30:22–5.
47. Iagaru A, Masamed R, Singer PA, et al. Detection of occult medullary thyroid cancer recurrence with 2-Deoxy-2-[F-18]fluoro-d-glucose-PET and PET/CT. Mol Imaging Biol 2007;9:72–7.
48. Adams S, Baum R, Rink T, et al. Limited value of fluorine-18 fluorodeoxyglucose positron emission tomography fort the imaging neuroendocrine tumors. Eur J Nucl Med 1998;25:79–83.
49. Okada J, Oonishi H, Yoshikawa K, et al. FDG-PET for predicting the prognosis of malignant lymphoma. Ann Nucl Med 1994;8:187–91.
50. Feine U, Lietzenmayer R, Hanke JP, et al. Fluorine-18-FDG and iodine-131-iodide uptake in thyroid cancer. J Nucl Med 1996;37:1468–72.
51. Musholt TJ, Musholt PB, Dehdashti F, et al. Evaluation of fluorodeoxyglucose-positron emission tomographic scanning and its association with glucose transporter expression in medullary thyroid carcinoma and pheochromocytoma: a clinical and molecular study. Surgery 1997;122:1049–60 [discussion: 1060–1].
52. Conti PS, Durski JM, Bacqai F, et al. Imaging of locally recurrent and metastatic thyroid cancer with positron emission tomography. Thyroid 1999;9:797–804.
53. Bergström M, Erikson B, Öberg K, et al. In vivo demonstration of enzyme activity in endocrine pancreatic tumors: decarboxylation of carbon-11-DOPA to carbon-11-dopamine. J Nucl Med 1996;37:32–7.
54. Pearse AG. The cytochemistry and ultrastructure of polypeptide hormone producing cells of APUD series and the embryologic, physiologic and pathologic implications of the concept. J Histochem Cytochem 1969;17:303–8.
55. Jager PL, Vaalburg W, Pruim J, et al. Radiolabelled amino acids: basic aspects and clinical applications in oncology. J Nucl Med 2001;42:432–5.
56. Ahlström H, Erikson B, Bergström M, et al. Pancreatic neuroendocrine tumors: diagnosis with PET. Radiology 1995;195:333–7.
57. Orlefors H, Sundin A, Ahsltröm H, et al. Positron emission tomography with 5-hydroxytriptophan in neuroendocrine tumors. J Clin Oncol 1998;16:2534–41.
58. Hoegerle S, Schneider B, Kraft A, et al. Imaging of a metastatic gastrointestinal carcinoid by F-18-DOPA positron emission tomography. Nuklearmedizin 1999;38:127–30.
59. Hoegerle S, Altehoefer C, Ghanem N, et al. F-18 DOPA positron emission tomography for tumor detection in patients with medullary thyroid carcinoma and elevated calcitonin levels. Eur J Nucl Med 2001;28:64–71.
60. Beuthien-Baumann B, Strumpf A, Zessin J, et al. Diagnostic impact of PET with 18F-FDG, 18F-DOPA and 3-O-methyl -6–18F-fluoro-DOPA in recurrent or metastatic medullary thyroid carcinoma. Eur J Nucl Med Mol Imaging 2007;34:1604–9.
61. Beuthien-Baumann B, Bredow J, Burchert W, et al. 3-O-methyl -6-18F-fluoro-L-DOPA and its evaluation in brain tumor imaging. Eur J Nucl Med Mol Imaging 2003;30:1004–8.
62. Feine U, Lietzenmayer R, Scheidhauer K, et al. Fluorine-18-FDG and iodine-131 uptake in thyroid cancer. J Nucl Med 1996;37:1468–72.
63. Gourgiotis L, Sarlis NJ, Reynolds JC, et al. Localization of medullary thyroid carcinoma metastasis in a multiple endocrine neoplasia type 2A patient by 6-F-18 fluorodopamine positron emission tomography. J Clin Endocrinol Metab 2003;88(2):637–41.
64. Oishi S, Sasaki M, Sato T, et al. Imaging and uptake mechanism of 131I-meta-iodobenzylguanidine in medullary thyroid carcinoma. Endocrinol Jpn 1986;33(3):309–15.

The Role of Iodine-124-Positron Emission Tomography Imaging in the Management of Patients with Thyroid Cancer

Ravinder K. Grewal, MD[a],*, Mark Lubberink, PhD[b],
Keith S. Pentlow, MSc[c], Steven M. Larson, MD[a]

KEYWORDS

- Iodine 124 • Dosimetry • Thyroid cancer

Molecular imaging is defined as imaging the key molecules or molecular-based events that underlie a physiologic or pathologic process.[1] For thyroid cancer, this approach includes imaging iodine transport by the sodium iodine transporter, which is active in about 80% of well-differentiated thyroid cancers. Iodine-124 imaging with positron emission tomography (I-124-PET) is ideal for this purpose because it provides high-resolution quantitative imaging data. Because iodine-131 is the mainstay for therapy in thyroid cancer, and because success or failure of therapy depends on the degree of iodine uptake, I-124-PET imaging can serve as a surrogate for this type of treatment.[2]

I-124 has a half-life of 4.2 days and a relatively complex decay scheme, with 22% of the disintegrations producing positrons of relatively high energies (1,532 keV and 2,135 keV), as well as a number of high-energy gamma and X-rays with energies as high as 1,691 keV. Despite the abundance of high-energy gamma photons, images with optimal quality can be generated and quantification of tracer uptake is achievable with this tracer. In 1960, Phillips and colleagues[3] demonstrated the use of I-124 in the treatment of thyroid carcinoma. Pentlow and colleagues[4,5] hypothesized that quantitative imaging with I-124 labeled antibodies appears to be feasible using a bismuth germanate (BGO)-based PET scanners. In a recent study comparing the image quality of different iodine isotopes (I-123, I-124, and I-131), I-124 gave the best imaging properties.[6] Not only does I-124 have superior sensitivity, but it also capable of estimating the functional volume of the thyroid tissue being examined.[7]

However, image quality and quantitative accuracy of PET imaging with I-124 are affected by the abundance of high-energy gamma rays and by the high energy of the positrons emitted, which lead to degradation of spatial resolution of the images generated.[8] In addition, in 50% of positron decays a coincident 602 keV gamma photon is also emitted, leading to possible "true coincidences" between one annihilation photon and the 602 keV gamma photon. This results in a quantitative bias

a Division of Nuclear Medicine, Department of Radiology, Memorial Sloan-Kettering Cancer Center, 1275 York Avenue, New York, NY 10065, USA
b Department of Nuclear Medicine and PET Research, VU University Medical Centre, PO Box 7057, 1007 MB Amsterdam, The Netherlands
c Nuclear Medicine Physics, Department of Medical Physics, Memorial Sloan-Kettering Cancer Center, 1275 York Avenue, New York, NY 10065, USA
* Corresponding author.
E-mail address: grewalr@mskcc.org (R.K. Grewal).

PET Clin 2 (2008) 313–320
doi:10.1016/j.cpet.2008.05.001
1556-8598/08/$ – see front matter © 2008 Elsevier Inc. All rights reserved.

in I-124-PET images, which has also been shown for other isotopes with similar decay schemes,[9–11] and corrections for this bias have been suggested. Because this bias is more or less uniformly distributed over the field of view of the scanner, its effect on quantification is small for a highly specific tracer such as I-124-iodide, but it is more important for I-124-labeled tracers with a homogeneous distribution throughout the body. The high abundance of gamma radiation in itself leads to increased detection of single photons, which in turn leads to increased random rates and, consequently, increased image noise. Simulation studies have shown that it is preferable to scan I-124 in three-dimensional (3D) mode because of down scatter of high energy photons in the lead or tungsten septa in conventional 2D mode and subsequent detection of these photons within the PET energy window.[12] Detection of photons with energy outside the scanner's energy window may also lead to inaccurate dead time correction.[10] A considerable improvement in clinical image quality was indeed achieved in 3D mode, especially by using a narrow energy window.[13] On state-of-the-art PET/CT systems, using dense detector materials such as lutetium oxyorthosilicate and lutetium yttrium oxyorthosilicate, the energy window is routinely narrower than that on BGO-based scanner. These crystals are also much faster than BGO, allowing for a shorter coincidence-timing window, which markedly decreases random coincidence rates. To date, however, no study has been published addressing the image quality and quantitative accuracy of I-124 imaging with 3D-only PET/CT systems. If I-124 is to be used for quantitative imaging aimed at dosimetry of I-131 therapy,

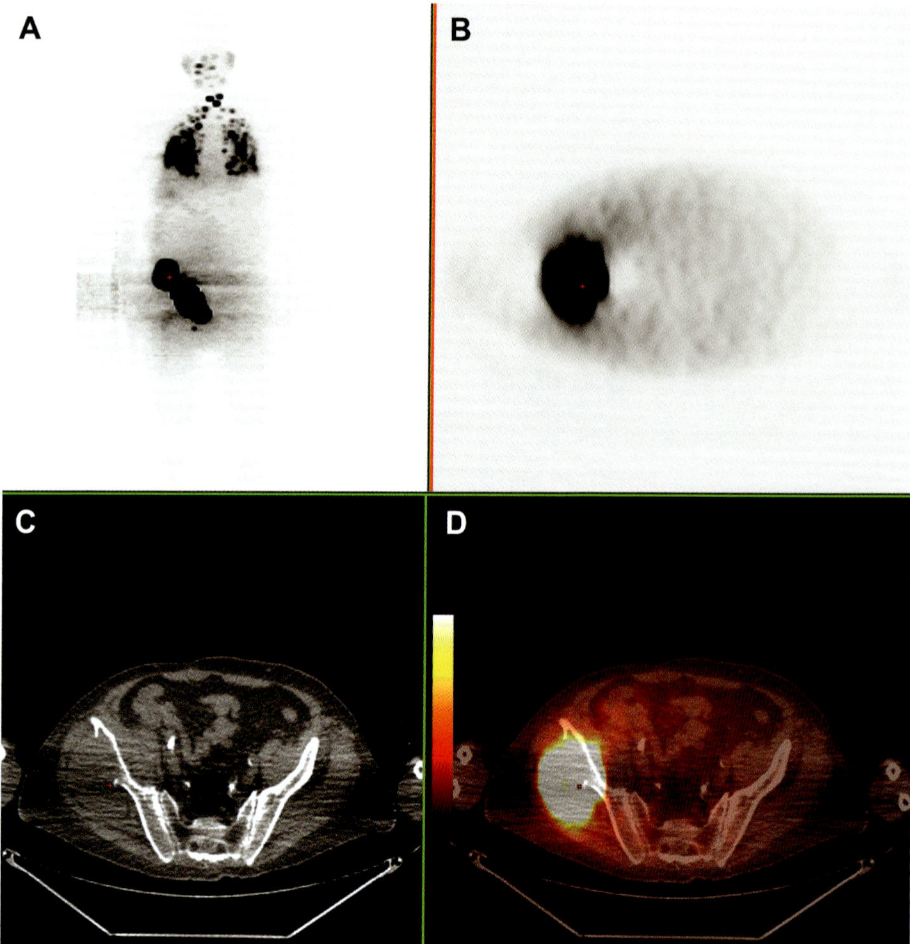

Fig. 1. Case 1 I-124 PET-CT scan (7.7 mCi baseline scan). (*A*) The maximum intensity projection (MIP) image at 48 hours shows iodine avid disease in the neck, bilateral lungs and right hemipelvis. The transaxial PET and CT images (*B*, *C*) or the fused PET/CT image (*D*) shows abnormal I-124 uptake in the lytic lesion involving the right iliac bone with extraosseous soft tissue component.

special interest should be given to the count rate linearity of the scanner, especially if PET imaging is done during therapy with I-131.

Despite these challenges, PET with I-124 provides images of high spatial and contrast resolutions when compared with conventional techniques. This results in detection of lesions with high sensitivity.[14] However, even with highly specific tracers like I-124, interpretation of PET images alone is difficult because of lack of anatomic correlate, thus making exact localization difficult.[15] PET/CT may overcome this deficiency. The combined PET/CT imaging provides coregistered PET and CT data to allow correlation of structural and functional imaging data, therefore improving management of patients with thyroid cancer and possibly other disorders.[16,17]

In a comparative study of 12 patients with differentiated thyroid cancer who were referred for diagnostic workup, lesion detectability was 100%, 87%, 83%, and 56% for combined I-124 PET/CT, I-124 PET alone, I-131 whole body scintigraphy (WBS), and CT, respectively. These findings indicate that I-124 PET/CT may provide incremental diagnostic value over the other imaging modalities.[14] These data also suggested that I-124 imaging can be performed 24 hours after radiotracer administration. Therefore, clinical decisions can be made much faster, as high-dose WBS with I-131 is usually performed 3 to 8 days after the administration of this tracer.

I-124 PET/CT is superior to I-131 WBS in detecting, localizing, and differentiating between the thyroid remnant and cervical lymph node metastases and distant metastases to the lungs, liver, adrenal gland, or bone marrow. In addition, the CT component of this technique can reveal iodine-negative metastatic lesions and, as a result, optimal treatment and management of the affected subjects can be achieved.[14]

Moreover, in patients who will be undergoing treatment with I-131 radioiodine therapy for thyroid cancer or thyrotoxicosis, I-124 PET imaging can be useful in providing absolute quantification, and therefore accurate dosimetry, of the administered therapeutic dose of I-131. A study by Eschmann and colleagues[18] determined the dosimetry of radioiodine therapy in 12 patients with toxic nodular goiters and 3 patients with differentiated thyroid cancer (two patients were referred for thyroid remnants ablation and the third one for treatment of multiple bone marrow metastases) by using I-124 PET. They were able to show that I-124 PET is helpful in volume

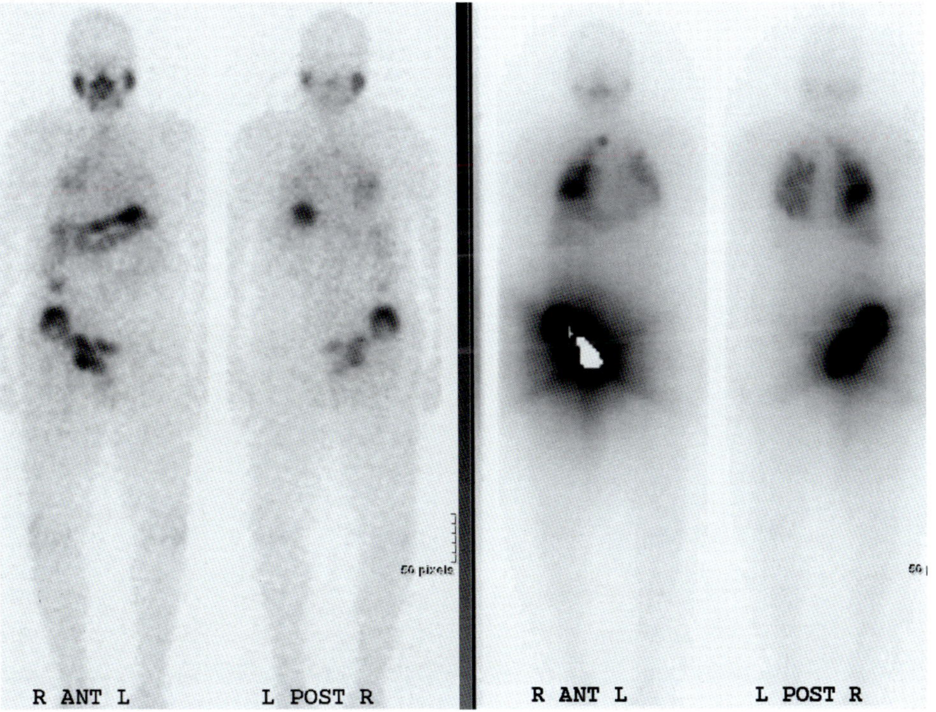

Fig. 2. Case 1 I-123 (diagnostic scan with 1.5 mCi) and I-131 (posttherapy scan after 150 mCi) whole body scans. Both studies demonstrate the radioactive iodine-avid disease in the lower neck, bilateral lung fields, and right hemipelvis.

estimations within an imprecision of approximately 20%, which they considered acceptable for clinical use. However, because of limited spatial resolution of this technique there is probably an overestimation of small nodular volumes, which could present a source of error for such lesions. Also, their results in three thyroid cancer patients showed that higher radiation doses were achieved in thyroid remnants than in metastatic disease and there was a considerable variability of the radiation doses delivered to the latter sites. They also predicted that in differentiated thyroid cancer metastases the radiation doses in the range of 70 Gy to 170 Gy would be delivered to the individual lesions.

The main advantage of I-124-PET imaging stems from its ability to predict lesional dosimetry, which would provide a scientific basis for determining the optimal dose for treatment with I-131.[17,18] This will result in achieving high therapeutic benefit by administering the maximum

dose of I-131 to the lesions, with acceptable toxicity to the body organs.[19]

Sgouros and colleagues[20] used a 3-dimensional-internal dosimetry (3D-ID) software and I-124-PET for retrospective lesion specific dosimetry in 15 subjects with metastatic thyroid carcinoma for I-131 therapy purposes. In this study, after the administration of the radiopharmaceutic, multiple PET images defined the spatial distribution of radioactivity at different time points. To process the reconstructed PET images for 3D-ID dosimetry calculations, they used the multiple mage analysis utility software package. This research demonstrated that there is substantial variability in intra- and intertumoral absorbed doses in individual patients, and a mean individual absorbed dose in the range of 1.2 Gy to 540 Gy was noted in this population.[21]

The first comprehensive study of normal organ dosimetry by I-124-PET imaging and 3D-ID software was performed by Kolbert and colleagues[22]

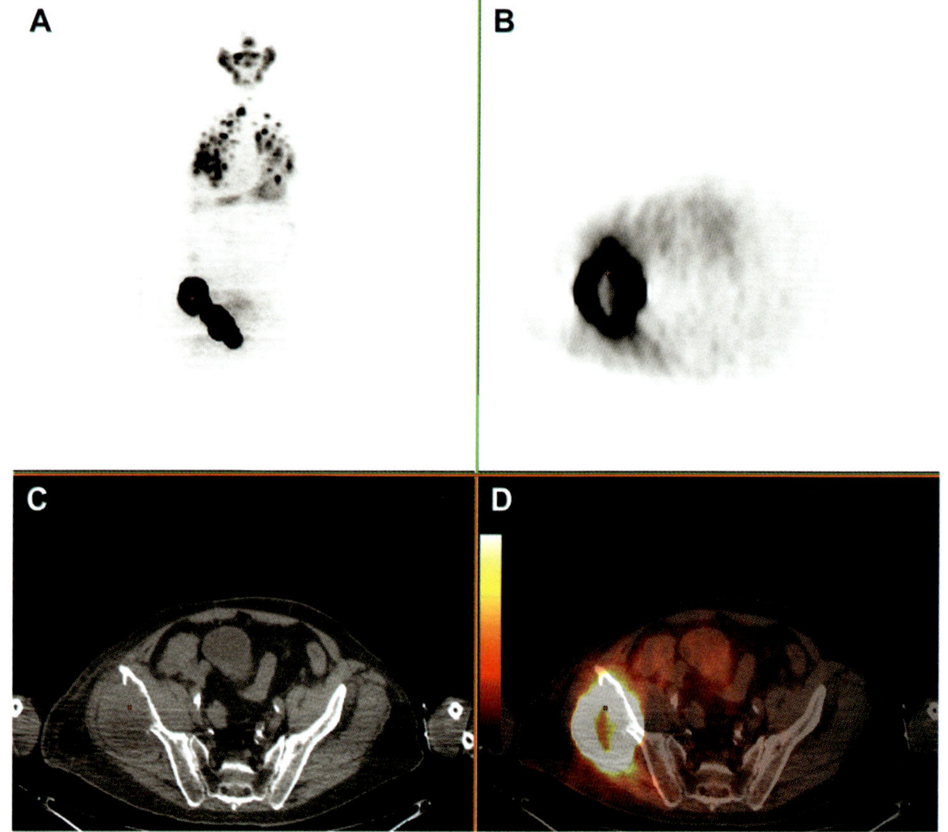

Fig. 3. Case 1 I-124 PET-CT scan (5.16 mCi follow-up study). (A) The MIP image at 48 hours again shows iodine-avid disease in the neck, bilateral lungs, and right hemipelvis. The transaxial PET and CT images (B, C) or the fused PET/CT image (D) shows abnormal I-124 uptake in the lytic lesion involving the right iliac bone with extraosseous soft tissue component.

in 26 thyroid cancer patients treated with I-131. Based on these data, the highest mean absorbed dose was noted in the right submandibular salivary gland and the lowest mean absorbed dose was seen in the brain.

In a recent study by Freudenberg and colleagues[23] in 28 consecutive thyroidectomized patients with high risk differentiated thyroid cancer, serial I-124-PET dosimetry was performed. The goal was to calculate the individualized I-131 therapy dose and determine absorbed lesion dose per GBq of administered I-131 activity so as to achieve a radiation dose of greater than or equal to 100 Gy to all metastases without exceeding 2 Gy to the blood. In addition, critical blood activity was calculated based on the blood and whole body counts. In this research, I-124-PET dosimetry changed the patient management in terms of therapeutic dose of I-131 administered in 25% of cases, and led to early multimodality

intervention in 32% of patients, compared with and relative to the standard empiric approaches. Another recent study of four pediatric patients ($\leq$18 years) with differentiated thyroid cancer, by Freudenberg and colleagues[24] showed that a standard adult I-124-PET/CT dosimetry protocol appears to be safe and informative in the pediatric age group. In this small study, disease management was modified or disease extent clarified in two out of four patients.

What follows are some case examples of thyroid cancer patients, with known metastatic disease, where I-124 dosimetry was considered to be of value for lesion-specific dosimetry.

CASE 1

An 86-year-old male, after investigation for laryngitis, was discovered to have right vocal cord paralysis and a 3.6-cm right thyroid lobe nodule. Fine

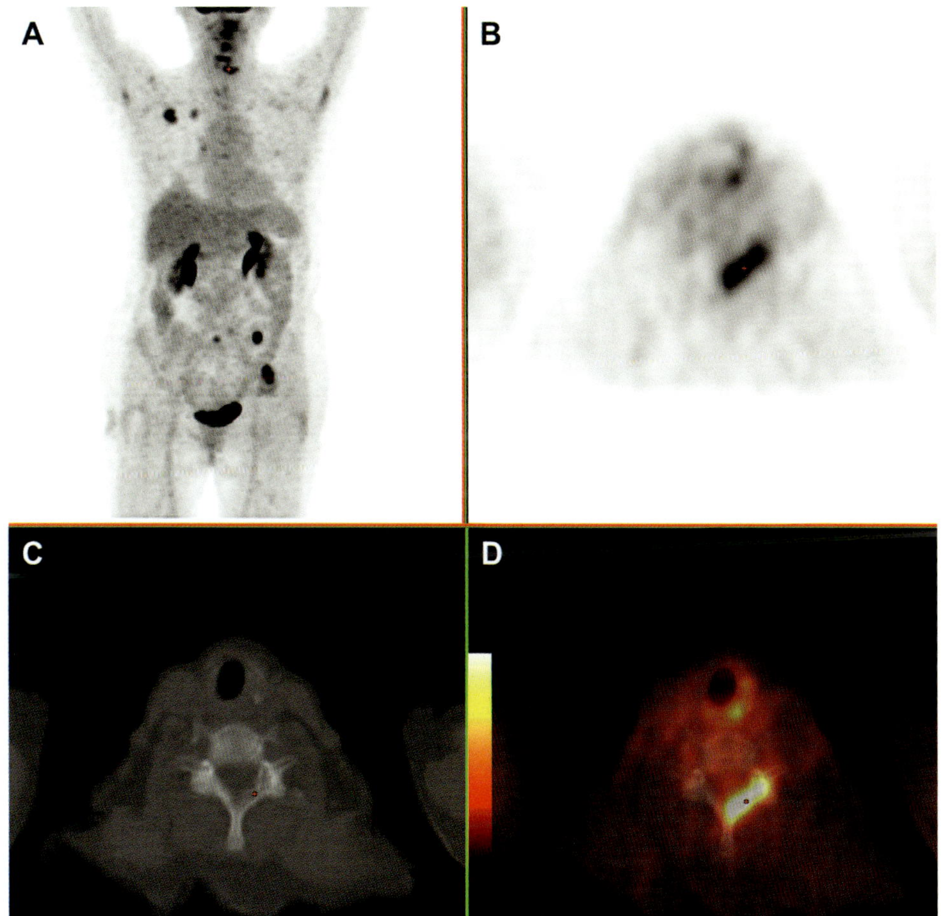

Fig. 4. Case 2 F-18 FDG PET-CT scan (15 mCi). (*A*) The MIP image shows FDG-avid disease in the neck, and osseous metastases in the spine, ribs, sacrum and left acetabulum. The transaxial PET and CT images (*B, C*) or the fused PET/CT image (*D*) shows abnormal FDG uptake in the lesion involving the left pedicle of C6 vertebra.

needle aspiration biopsy revealed a suspicious follicular lesion. Subsequent PET-CT scanning demonstrated 18 fluorodeoxyglucose (FDG) activity in the right thyroid nodule, pulmonary lesions, and bone marrow metastases in the right hemipelvis. Biopsy of a right pelvic lesion confirmed metastatic thyroid carcinoma. Total thyroidectomy was performed. Pathology showed a poorly differentiated thyroid carcinoma, predominantly of insular subtype. There was extensive tumor necrosis in the right thyroid lobe, significant capsular and blood vessel invasion, which included invasion of medium-sized extrathyroidal vasculature. Perithyroid fibroadipose tissue was infiltrated by the cancer cells and the tumor extended close to the inked margin. Esophageal wall margin biopsy also revealed poorly differentiated thyroid carcinoma. Subsequently, the patient received palliative radiotherapy to the right pelvic metastasis. He was then referred for I-124 dosimetry. I-124 was obtained as a unit dose from a regional vendor in the form of an oral solution. Seven mCi of I-124 were administered orally and the patient was scanned at 4, 24, 72, and 144 hours on a GE Discovery STE PET scanner. Using the Medical Internal Radiation Committee methodology, the measured concentration in the lesions over time was used to calculate radiation absorbed dose. The I-124-PET scan at 48 hours showed metastatic disease in the neck, lungs, and right hemipelvis (**Fig. 1**). The pelvic lesion demonstrated very nonuniform uptake, with a maximum of 3.06 kBq/mL per MBq administered (3.06 µCi/mL per mCi administered). Accordingly, while some parts of this lesion had a predicted mean absorbed dose for I-131 of 92 Gy per GBq (340 rads/mCi), resulting in a maximum dose of 420 Gy (42,000 rads) for the subsequent therapy dose of 120 mCi, much of the lesion appeared to receive considerably lower radiation. The other lesions were in the range of 5% to 10% of this maximum value. The after-therapy scan demonstrated metastatic disease in the neck, lungs, and right hemipelvis (**Fig. 2**). After 6 months the patient underwent a follow up repeat I-124 dosimetry to estimate the relationship between the radiation dose delivered and response to in the metastatic lesions following the therapeutic administration of I-131 (**Fig. 3**). The degree of uptake in areas previously noted to be positive was reduced, but adjacent new sites of uptake were seen.

CASE 2

A 72-year-old female with metastatic follicular thyroid carcinoma was discovered to have a skull nodule. Biopsy was consistent with follicular thyroid cancer. Thereafter, CT showed a large calcified thyroid mass and lower thoracic vertebral metastasis causing cord compression. The patient underwent external beam radiotherapy to the vertebral spine followed by excision of the skull metastasis and total thyroidectomy. Pathology revealed a 10.5 cm moderately differentiated, widely invasive follicular thyroid cancer with multiple positive lymph nodes. In September 2002, she received 125-mCi I-131. After therapy scan showed multiple bone marrow metastases. Follow-up therapy with 414-mCi I-131 in February 2003 again revealed multiple skeletal lesions. In October 2003 she received 420-mCi I-131, and after therapy scan showed foci of uptake in the right chest, lower thoracic spine, pelvis, and no clear-cut abnormality. The patient was treated with 421-mCi of I-131 in June 2004 and after therapy scan showed activity in the right posterior skull, right lower chest, lower thoracic spine, right and left pelvis, and right proximal femur. FDG-PET scan in September 2005 showed local recurrent disease in the neck and osseous metastases in the sacrum, left ilium, C-spine, ribs, right distal clavicle, sternal notch, and skull (**Fig. 4**). The patient was then referred for I-124 dosimetry. The 48-hour I-124-PET scan (**Fig. 5**) showed foci of abnormal radiotracer uptake in the left mastoid region, right occipital skull, lower C-spine, T12,

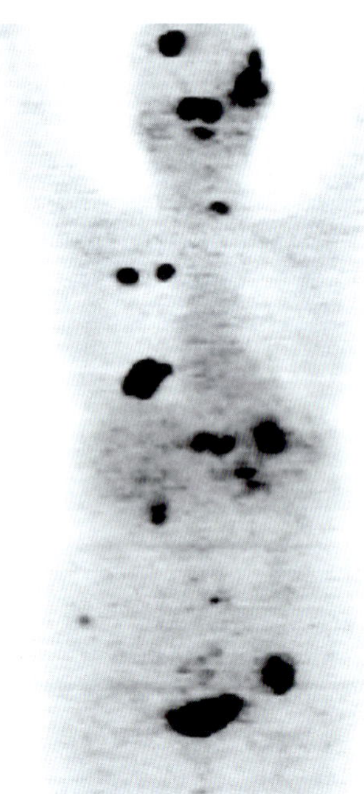

Fig. 5. Case 2 I-124 PET-CT scan (6 mCi). The MIP image at 48 hours shows iodine-avid disease in the skull, spine, right upper and lower ribs, sacrum, left acetabulum, and right iliac bone.

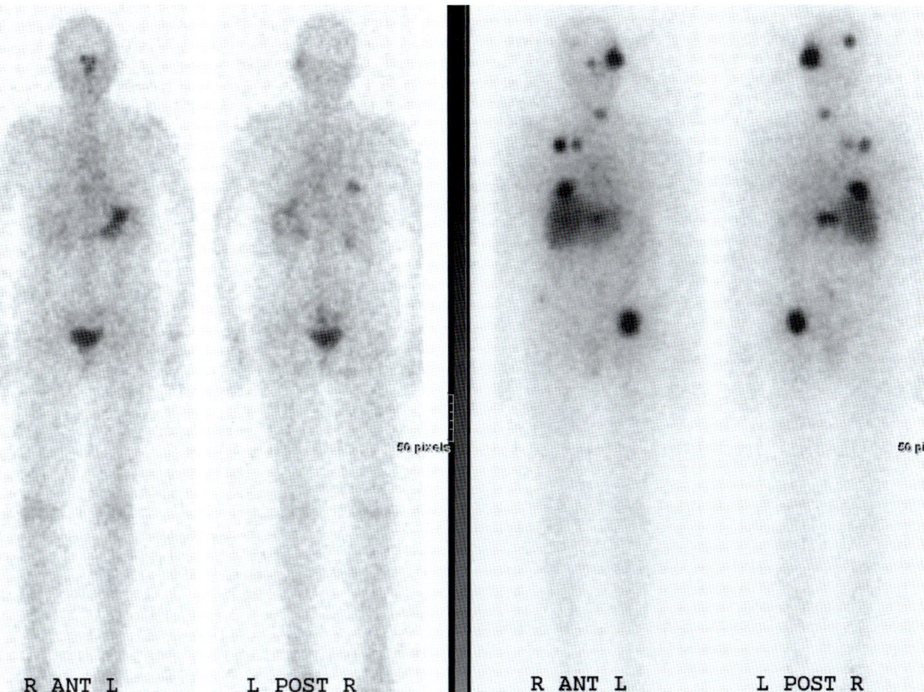

Fig. 6. Case 2 I-123 (diagnostic scan with 1.5 mCi) and I-131 (posttherapy scan after 320 mCi) whole body scans. The I-123 scan shows faint foci of uptake in the skull, right posterior chest and right proximal femur. The I-131 post therapy scan demonstrates radioactive iodine-avid disease in skull, spine, right upper and lower ribs, sacrum, left acetabulum, and right iliac bone.

right upper anterior ribs, right posterior rib, sacrum, left acetabulum, and right iliac bone. There was symmetrically increased radiotracer uptake in the region of the frontal/ethmoid sinuses, possibly because of inflammatory lesions or metastatic disease. Physiologic radiotracer accumulation was seen in the salivary glands, stomach, bowel, kidneys and urinary bladder. The maximum tolerated activity was calculated to be 670 mCi. The maximum uptake (in the left mastoid lesion) was only 0.11 kBq/mL per MBq administered (0.11 µCi/mL per mCi administered). This yielded a predicted mean absorbed dose for 131-I of 3.1 Gy per GBq (11.3 rads/mCi), resulting in a maximum dose of 36 Gy (3,600 rads) for the subsequent therapy dose of 321 mCi. The other lesions were in the range of 10% to 25% of this maximum value. The I-123 diagnostic scan (**Fig. 6**) showed subtle foci of uptake in skull, spine, right posterior chest, and left acetabular region. The after-therapy scan showed iodine-avid osseous metastases in the skull, ribs, spine, and bony pelvis (see **Fig. 6**).

SUMMARY AND FUTURE DIRECTIONS

I-124 PET dosimetry provides accurate quantification of radiation absorbed doses to thyroid cancer and metastatic disease in the body. In addition, I-124 has been used to label various carriers, such as antibodies, peptides, amino acids, and reporter genes.[25] It has been shown that I-124 PET/CT, as a probe for assessing sodium iodide symporter (NIS) in animal models, allows the tracking of stably transfected or intravenously transfected tumors. This technique provides accurate and noninvasive imaging tools for visualizing the distribution and gene expression of a replicating viral vector in living systems.[26] I-124 labeled annexin-V is used in imaging apoptosis, which is an important pathogenic mechanism in many diseases, including cancer, and provides valuable information regarding the response to therapeutic intervention.[27,28] In addition, I-124 meta-iodobenzylguanidine can be useful in imaging of medullary thyroid cancer.

REFERENCES

1. Mankoff DA. A definition of molecular imaging. J Nucl Med 2007;48:18N, 21N.
2. Erdi YE, Macapinlac H, Larson SM, et al. Radiation dose assessment for I-131 therapy of thyroid cancer using I-124 PET imaging. Clin Positron Imaging 1999;2:41–6.

3. Phillips AF, Haybittle JL, Newbery GR. Use of Iodine-124 for the treatment of carcinoma of the thyroid. Acta Unio Int Contra Cancrum 1960;16:1434–8.

4. Pentlow KS, Graham MC, Lambrecht RM, et al. Quantitative imaging of I-124 using positron emission tomography with applications to radioimmuno-diagnosis and radioimmunotherapy. Med Phys 1991;18:357–66.

5. Pentlow KS, Graham MC, Lambrecht RM, et al. Quantitative imaging of iodine-124 with PET. J Nucl Med 1996;37:1557–62.

6. Rault E, Vandenberghe S, Van Holen R, et al. Comparison of image quality of different iodine isotopes (I-123, I-124, and I-131). Cancer Biother Radiopharm 2007;22:423–30.

7. Glaser M, Luthra SK, Brady F. Applications of positron-emitting halogens in PET oncology (Review). Int J Oncol 2003;22:253–67.

8. Herzog H, Tellman L, Qaim SM, et al. PET quantitation and imaging of the non-pure positron-emitting iodine isotope 124I. Appl Radiat Isot 2002;56:673–9.

9. Pentlow KS, Finn RD, Larson SM, et al. Quantitative imaging of Yttrium-86 with PET. The occurrence and correction of anomalous apparent activity in high density regions. Clin Positron Imaging 2000;3: 85–90.

10. Lubberink M, Schneider H, Bergstrom M, et al. Quantitative imaging and correction for cascade gamma radiation of 76Br with 2D and 3D PET. Phys Med Biol 2002;47:3519–34.

11. Beattie BJ, Finn RD, Rowland DJ, et al. Quantitative imaging of bromine-76 and yttrium-86 with PET: a method for the removal of spurious activity introduced by cascade gamma rays. Med Phys 2003; 30:2410–23.

12. Kolthammer J, Salem N, Fiedler K, et al. Downscatter contamination from high-energy photons of I-124 in 2D and 3D PET. IEEE 2004. Nuclear Science Symposium Conference record 2004;3629–33.

13. Lubberink M, van Schie A, de Jong HW, et al. Acquisition settings for PET of 124-I administered simultaneously with therapeutic amounts of 131I. J Nucl Med 2006;47:1375–81.

14. Freudenberg LS, Antoch G, Jentzen W, et al. Value of I-124-PET/CT in staging of patients with differentiated thyroid cancer. Eur Radiol 2004;14:2092–8.

15. Beyer T, Townsend DW, Brun T, et al. A combined PET/CT scanner for clinical oncology. J Nucl Med 2000;41:1369–79.

16. Freudenberg LS, Antoch G, Gorges R, et al. Combined PET/CT with iodine-124 in diagnosis of spread metastatic thyroid carcinoma: a case report. Eur Radiol 2003;13:L19–23.

17. Larson SM, Robbins R. Positron emission tomography in thyroid cancer management. Semin Roentgenol 2002;37:169–74.

18. Eschmann SM, Reischl G, Bilger K, et al. Evaluation of dosimetry of radioiodine therapy in benign and malignant thyroid disorders by means of iodine-124 and PET. Eur J Nucl Med Mol Imaging 2002; 29:760–7.

19. Dorn R, Kopp J, Vogt H, et al. Dosimetry-guided radioactive iodine treatment in patients with metastatic differentiated thyroid cancer: Largest safe dose using a risk-adapted approach. J Nucl Med 2003;44:451–6.

20. Sgouros G, Kolbert KS, Sheikh A, et al. Patient-specific dosimetry for I-131 thyroid cancer therapy using I-124 PET and 3-dimensional-internal dosimetry (3D-ID) software. J Nucl Med 2004;45:1366–72.

21. Kolbert KS, Sgouros G. Display and manipulation of SPECT and CT studies for radiolabeled antibody therapy [Abstract]. Cancer Biother Radiopharm 1998;302.

22. Kolbert KS, Pentlow KS, Pearson JR, et al. Prediction of absorbed dose to normal organs in thyroid cancer patients treated with I-131 by use of I-124 PET and 3-dimensional internal dosimetry software. J Nucl Med 2007;48:143–9.

23. Freudenberg LS, Jentzen W, Gorges R, et al. I-124-PET dosimetry in advanced differentiated thyroid cancer: Therapeutic impact. Nuklearmedizin 2007; 46:121–8.

24. Freudenberg LS, Jentzen W, Marlowe RJ, et al. 124-iodine positron emission tomography/computed tomography dosimetry in pediatric patients with differentiated thyroid cancer. Exp Clin Endocrinol Diabetes 2007;115:690–3.

25. Van Nostrand D. New approaches in nuclear medicine for thyroid cancer. Totowa (NJ): Humana Press; 2006.

26. Dingli D, Kemp BJ, O'Connor MK, et al. Combined I-124 positron emission tomography/computed tomography imaging of NIS gene expression in animal models of stably transfected and intravenously transfected tumor. Mol Imaging Biol 2006;8:16–23.

27. Keen HG, Dekker BA, Disley L, et al. Imaging apoptosis in vivo using 124I-annexin V and PET. Nucl Med Biol 2005;32:395–402.

28. Dekker B, Keen H, Lyons S, et al. MBP-annexin V radiolabeled directly with iodine-124 can be used to image apoptosis in vivo using PET. Nucl Med Biol 2005;32:241–52.

Clinical Significance of Incidental Focal Versus Diffuse Thyroid Uptake on FDG-PET Imaging

Wengen Chen, MD, PhD[a], Geming Li, MD[a], Molly Parsons, BA[a], Hongming Zhuang, MD, PhD[a,b], Abass Alavi, MD, PhD[a,*]

KEYWORDS

- FDG-PET • Thyroid • Incidental uptake

[18]F-Fluorodeoxyglucose (FDG) positron emission tomography (PET) and PET/CT have been widely used in the evaluation of various pathologic processes, including malignancies[1,2] and infection/inflammation.[3,4] FDG accumulation in normal thyroid tissue is usually low or absent, as noted on the whole body FDG-PET scan.[5] Occasionally, diffusely or focally increased FDG uptake can be detected as an incidental finding in the thyroid. As a consequence of the increasing use of whole body FDG-PET scan in clinical practice, frequently incidental focal or diffuse FDG uptake in the thyroid is being noted. Accurate interpretation of these unexpected findings remains a challenge for nuclear medicine physicians or radiologists. In most settings, an appropriate decision process presents a dilemma for referring physicians. Because of the relatively recent introduction of FDG-PET to the daily practice of medicine, there are still no established criteria for the diagnosis of malignancy based on incidental lesions noted on the scan. In this article we review the prevalence of incidental FDG uptake in the thyroid gland as seen on PET scan and the differential diagnosis, including the risk for malignancy of such lesions. The role of uptake patterns and the role of standardized uptake values (SUVs) in differentiating between malignant and benign lesions are also discussed.

PREVALENCE OF INCIDENTAL THYROID UPTAKE ON FLUORODEOXYGLUCOSE POSITRON EMISSION TOMOGRAPHY SCAN

In earlier reports, thyroid FDG uptake was considered as normal variance.[6,7] This conclusion was purely an assumption, however, because in most settings no biochemical or histologic data were available to support the basis for this interpretation. Incidental thyroid lesions are usually defined as newly identified thyroid abnormalities encountered during routine imaging studies such as ultrasonography (US), CT, or MR imaging for unrelated diseases.[8] With the advent of FDG-PET and its proven role for assessing a variety of malignancies, great interest has arisen about the significance of incidental FDG uptake in the thyroid and the need for optimal management of patients with these findings. FDG uptake in the thyroid falls into two distinct patterns: diffuse (**Fig. 1**) or focal (**Fig. 2**). The prevalence and rate of malignancy in patients with abnormal FDG uptake differ substantially from those detected by other modalities, such as US.

The prevalence of incidental thyroid FDG uptake on PET, including focal and diffuse uptake, ranges from 1.8% to 2.9% in most of the large-scale retrospective studies published to date (**Table 1**). In 2001, Cohen and colleagues[9] reported 102 cases of incidental thyroid FDG uptake in 4525

[a] Division of Nuclear Medicine, Department of Radiology, Hospital of the University of Pennsylvania, University of Pennsylvania School of Medicine, 110 Donner, 3400 Spruce Street, Philadelphia, PA 19104, USA
[b] Division of Nuclear Medicine, Department of Radiology, The Children's Hospital of Philadelphia, University of Pennsylvania School of Medicine, South 34th Street, Philadelphia, PA 19104, USA
* Corresponding author.
E-mail address: abass.alavi@uphs.upenn.edu (A. Alavi).

PET Clin 2 (2008) 321–329
doi:10.1016/j.cpet.2008.04.001

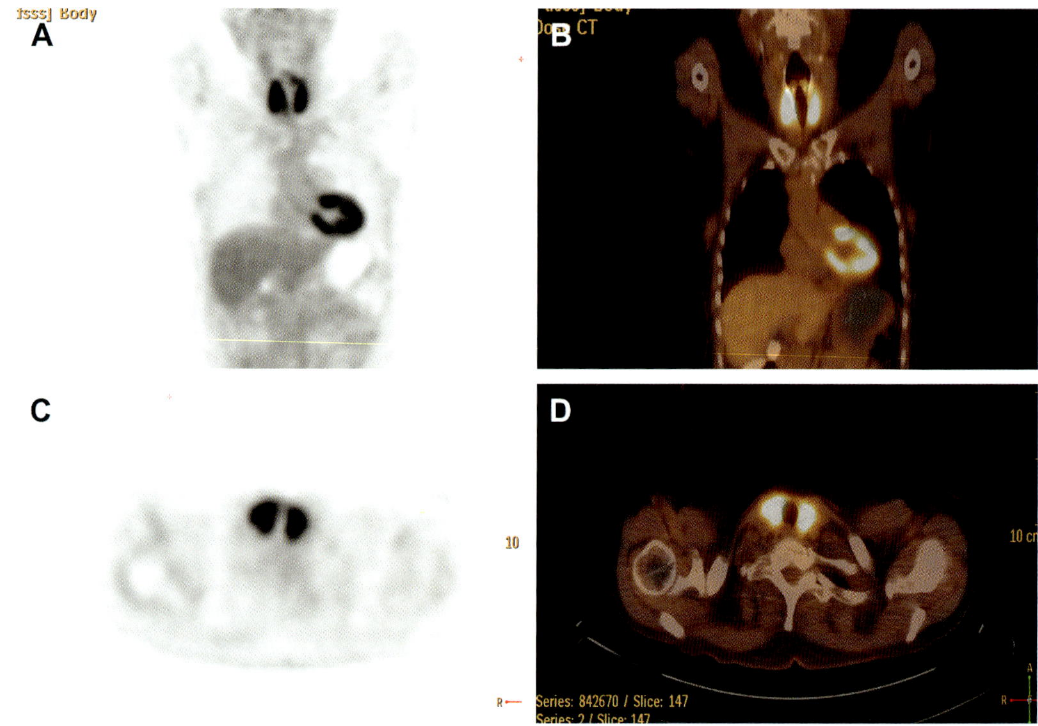

Fig. 1. FDG-PET/CT coronal (*A*, PET; *B*, fused) and transaxial scans (*C*, PET; *D*, fused) of a 65-year-old woman with cervical cancer demonstrate diffuse FDG uptake (SUV$_{max}$ = 8.5) in both lobes of the thyroid gland.

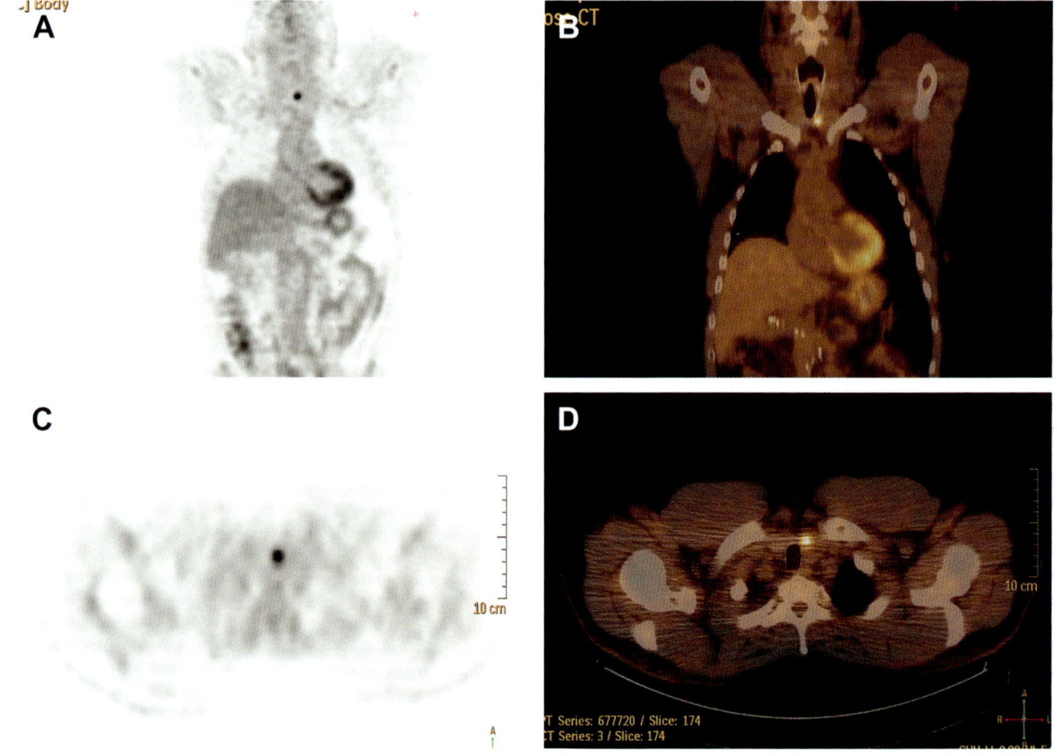

Fig. 2. FDG-PET/CT coronal (*A*, PET; *B*, fused) and transaxial scans (*C*, PET; *D*, fused) of a 52-year-old man with pancreatic cancer demonstrate a focal FDG uptake in the inferior pole of the left thyroid (SUV$_{max}$ = 6.0).

patients (2.3%) who had undergone PET examination for staging purposes for other cancers. Uptake among these 102 cases was focal in 71 (70%) and diffuse in 31 (30%). Similarly, Kang and colleagues[10] reported a prevalence of 2.2% (29/1330) with 72% focal (21/29) and 28% diffuse uptakes (8/29). In a study published by Kim and colleagues,[11] the prevalence was 2.2% (90/4136); half (45/90) had focal and half (45/90) had diffuse uptakes. Recently, Are and colleagues[12] identified 263 cases of incidental thyroid FDG uptake in 8800 patients with a prevalence of 2.9% (263/8800), of which 38% (101/263) were focal and 62% (162/263) were diffuse.

Other authors focused only on the prevalence of focal thyroid FDG uptake alone or diffuse uptake alone in patients undergoing a PET scan and showed relatively variable results (**Table 2**). For example, Chen and colleagues[13] and Chu and colleagues[14] noted a prevalence of 1.2% for focal thyroid FDG uptake only (diffuse uptake cases were excluded from analysis), which is close to the incidence of 1.8% to 2.9%, by including focal and diffuse uptake mentioned previously by assuming that focal and diffuse uptakes appear with equal frequency based on evidence from the reported studies. Bogsrud and colleagues[15] recently reported a prevalence of 1.1% with focal uptake (79/7347), whereas in a study by Choi and colleagues[16] in 2006, a much higher prevalence of 4.0% of focal thyroid uptake was noticed in a population of 1763 patients. Yi and colleagues[17] also reported a prevalence of 4.3% (6/140) of focal thyroid FDG uptake. Recently in a retrospective study, Nam and colleagues[18] noted a prevalence of 2.8% (19/689) with focal uptake, which is also higher than others. In contrast, a low prevalence of focal thyroid FDG uptake has been noticed. In a recent study by King and colleagues,[19] 22 cases of focal thyroid uptake were identified from a total of 15,711 cases with a prevalence of only 0.1%. The authors believe that their low prevalence may be related to a selection bias because the cases were solely from a melanoma center and most of their patients had a single malignancy (melanoma), which is different from other studies in which the targeted population was diverse.

Several studies have examined the prevalence of diffuse thyroid uptake alone. In 1998, Yasuda and colleagues[20] identified 36 cases of diffuse thyroid uptake among 1102 patients (3.2%) who had undergone a PET scan. Recently, Karantanis and colleagues[21] showed a prevalence of 2.9% with diffuse thyroid uptake (138/4732). Both studies showed a higher prevalence of diffuse thyroid FDG uptake compared with that reported in the large-scale studies mentioned

previously. A study published by Kurata and colleagues[22] showed a prevalence of 1.5% (25/1626) with diffuse thyroid uptake, however.

It is important to note that the target populations in most of these studies were cancer patients who had PET scan for staging or restaging, except for two studies in which PET was performed in healthy subjects undergoing cancer screening. Of the latter two studies, one was published by Chen and colleagues[13] in 2005 in which a prevalence of 1.2% of focal thyroid uptake rate was shown in 4803 healthy subjects. The other was published by Kang and colleagues[10] in which the population (1330) contained cancer patients ($n = 999$) and healthy subjects ($n = 331$). No significant difference was found in the prevalence of thyroid FDG uptake between the two groups.

Based on the data in the literature, it is reasonable to propose that in cancer patients or healthy individuals who undergo PET scan, the prevalence of incidental thyroid FDG uptake is approximately 2% to 3%, with approximately half demonstrating focal and the other half demonstrating diffuse uptake pattern. The prevalence of incidental thyroid FDG uptake on PET scan is much lower than that reported on US studies, which is approximately 19% to 46% in the general population.[23] Risk of a malignant process in patients with the incidental thyroid uptake on PET is much higher in the FDG-PET population than that of the US group, however, which suggests a higher clinical significance of incidental thyroid uptake on the PET scans.

PREVALENCE OF MALIGNANCY OF INCIDENTAL THYROID UPTAKE ON FLUORODEOXYGLUCOSE POSITRON EMISSION TOMOGRAPHY SCAN

The risk of malignancy associated with diffuse and focal thyroid FDG uptake is different. Diffuse thyroid FDG uptake is most commonly benign and is usually caused by chronic lymphocytic (Hashimoto's) thyroiditis. Of the 36 diffuse thyroid FDG uptake cases identified from 1102 patients by Yasuda and colleagues,[20] all were found to be caused by thyroiditis. Karantanis and colleagues[21] showed that all 138 cases with diffuse uptake among the 4732 patients were also caused by thyroiditis. Similar results were noted in other studies.[9–12] In a few cases, diffuse thyroid FDG uptake was also linked to Graves' disease.[24,25] In the population reported in the literature to date, only two cases of diffuse thyroid FDG uptake were caused by malignancy: one case harbored a papillary carcinoma associated with Hashimoto's thyroiditis,[22] and the other case showed metastasis from lung cancer.[12]

Table 1
Prevalence and malignancy of incidental focal and diffuse thyroid fluorodeoxyglucose uptake in representative studies

Author	Year	Number of Patients	Prevalence			Malignancy of Focal Uptake (%)
			Total (%)	Focal (%)	Diffuse (%)	
Cohen and colleagues[9]	2001	4525	102 (2.3)	71 (1.6)	31 (0.7)	7/14 (50)
Kang and colleagues[10]	2003	1330	29 (2.2)	21 (1.6)	8 (0.6)	4/15 (27)
Kim and colleagues[11]	2005	4136	90 (2.2)	45 (1.1)	45 (1.1)	16/32 (50)
Are and colleagues[12]	2007	8800	263 (2.9)	101 (1.1)	162 (1.8)	24/57 (42)
Kurata and colleagues[22]	2007	1626	29 (1.8)	4 (0.3)	25 (1.5)	2/4 (50)

Table 2
Prevalence and malignancy of incidental focal thyroid fluorodeoxyglucose uptake in representative studies

Author	Year	Number of Patients	Prevalence (%)	Risk of Malignancy (%)
Chen and colleagues[13]	2005	4803	60 (1.2)	7/50 (14)
Yi and colleagues[17]	2005	140	6 (4.3)	4/7 (57)
Choi and colleagues[16]	2006	1763	70 (4.0)	17/44 (39)
Chu and colleagues[14]	2006	6241	76 (1.2)	4/14 (29)
King and colleagues[19]	2007	15,711	22 (0.1)	3/21 (14)
Bogsrud and colleagues[15]	2007	7347	79 (1.1)	17/48 (35)
Nam and colleagues[18]	2007	689	19 (2.8)	5/12 (42)

Focal uptake lesions in the thyroid, on the other hand, have a significant incidence of being malignant (**Tables 1** and **2**). In a series by Cohen and colleagues[9] of 14 patients with focal FDG uptake with final thyroid biopsy results, 7 (50%) had thyroid cancer, 6 had nodular hyperplasia, and one had thyroiditis. Cytologic diagnosis was available in 32 of 45 focal thyroid lesions reported by Kim and colleagues,[11] which revealed 14 papillary carcinomas and 2 follicular carcinomas for a total of 16 malignancies (50%). In a recent study by Are and colleagues,[12] 24 of 57 patients were found to have malignancies, indicating a 42% probability of malignancy. Nam and colleagues[18] found that 5 of 12 cases with focal lesions were malignant. Similar high risks for cancer have been noted in several case reports in the literature. For example, of the eight patients with thyroid lesions detected incidentally on whole-body PET scan in the study by Van den Bruel and colleagues,[26] seven patients underwent surgery. They reported three papillary thyroid carcinomas, two medullary thyroid carcinomas, and two follicular adenomas in this group. These results indicated a 63% malignancy rate. In a study by Yi and colleagues[17] of seven patients who had incidental thyroid lesions, four had lesions that were pathologically confirmed to be papillary thyroid carcinoma and one had a lesion that was benign at thyroidectomy. The remaining two patients had no histology results because of inability to visualize a specific target to biopsy on CT or US. These findings correspond to a malignancy rate of 57% (4/7). In a case report by Davis and colleagues,[27] all five cases of focal FDG uptake were finally diagnosed as papillary carcinomas.

A relatively lower risk was reported in other large series. A recent study by Chu and colleagues[14] detected 76 incidental findings in the thyroid gland; 14 patients underwent fine needle aspiration biopsy and 1 had a thyroid lobectomy. Papillary thyroid carcinoma was found in four (29%) of the specimens examined. Kang and colleagues[10] noted that 4 of 15 (27%) incidental findings were positive for thyroid cancer. Of the 60 patients who had thyroid incidental findings reported by Chen and colleagues,[13] 50 underwent US fine needle aspiration, which revealed 43 benign lesions and 7 papillary carcinomas with a 14% malignancy rate. In the study by Bogsrud and colleagues[15] in 2007, of the 48 patients who had histologic diagnosis, 17 had malignancy with a risk of 35%: papillary thyroid carcinoma in 12 patients, cytologic suspicious follicular carcinoma in 2, metastasis from squamous cell carcinoma in 1, and lymphoma in 2.

Occasionally, a thyroid lesion with focally and diffusely increased FDG uptake is seen on whole-body PET scans (**Fig. 3**). The significance of this type of lesion is not clear. Choi and colleagues[16] reported that five subjects with diffuse and focal uptake had no malignancy. In a study by Kurata and colleagues,[22] of the four subjects with focal plus diffuse FDG uptake, two had papillary carcinoma associated with Hashimoto's thyroiditis, and the remaining two had adenomatous goiter associated with Hashimoto's thyroiditis. Based on these results, it is appropriate to treat a mixed pattern of focal and diffuse uptake as focal uptake.

Based on the retrospective nature of the studies, the accurate rate of malignancy in this population cannot be determined. According to the data available, however, it is acceptable to conclude that the estimated risk of malignancy for focal thyroid FDG uptake on PET scan is approximately 30% to 50%. Most of these cases are primary thyroid carcinoma, particularly papillary type, with a few cases of primary lymphoma or metastasis from other malignancies. Metastatic thyroid

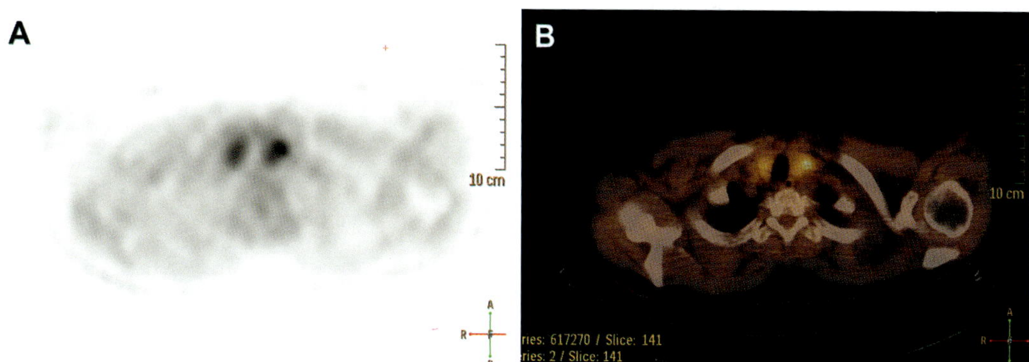

Fig. 3. FDG-PET/CT transaxial scans (*A*, PET; *B*, fused) of a 72-year-old woman with bilateral breast cancer demonstrate combined diffuse FDG uptake in the entire thyroid gland and a focal uptake in the left thyroid lobe.

cancer is rare, accounting for less than 1% of cases of thyroid malignancy in most clinical series.[28,29] Focal thyroid FDG uptake incidentally detected in patients who have cancer and are undergoing PET scan for staging and other purposes should not be considered as metastasis from the known primary cancer without histologic confirmation.

The 30% to 50% risk of malignancy in focal thyroid FDG uptake incidentally noted is much higher than that of the 4% to 12.6% risk in nodules detected by the US examination.[23] The difference may be caused by the fact that FDG-PET is a functional imaging modality. This finding may not report the incidence in the general population because most subjects who undergo a PET scan are known to have cancer and may be at high risk for other cancers. It is known that the coexistence of two or more different types of malignancy is not uncommon in patients who are genetically predisposed to cancer. Dong and Hemminki[30] reported that 8.5% of 633,964 patients with known cancers were subsequently proven to have other previously unrecognized primary cancers. Ueno and colleagues[31] showed that 5.2% of 24,498 patients who had cancer had multiple cancers. This phenomenon may be explained by the fact that some cancers tend to share the same risk factors or that subsequent cancers may be a result of potentially carcinogenic effects of the treatment of the initial malignancy, such as radiation therapy, chemotherapy, or both.

In the series discussed previously, only a small fraction of patients with incidental thyroid FDG uptake had histologic diagnosis of the underlying process. In most patients, the extent and severity of the primary disease did not justify further investigation of the incidental thyroid uptake, which was considered somewhat irrelevant to the management of the patient.

ROLE OF UPTAKE PATTERNS AND STANDARDIZED UPTAKE VALUES IN DIFFERENTIATING CANCER FROM BENIGN DISORDERS

The uptake patterns of FDG in the gland are considered significant in differentiating between malignant and benign processes. Most patients with diffuse uptake suffer from benign thyroiditis. Focal lesions harbor a relatively high risk for malignancy of approximately 30% to 50%. It is important to develop the means to distinguish between malignant and benign disorders in focal lesions.

The value of SUVs for differentiating between malignant and benign tumors of the thyroid on PET scan is still controversial. Some authors have suggested that SUVs may be of value for this purpose.[9,10,13,16] For example, Cohen and colleagues[9] noted that in 15 patients who had pathologic diagnosis of the underlying disease, the average SUV was higher in malignant lesions (6.92 ± 1.54) compared with that of benign lesions (3.37 ± 0.21). In contrast, others have shown no difference of SUV between the two groups, with significant overlap of SUV among different lesions.[11,18,32] Two studies showed that neither maximum nor average SUV could distinguish accurately between benign and malignant lesions in cases of focal thyroid FDG uptake.[11,12]

The varying results about the SUV of malignant and benign lesions could be related to the following: the partial volume effect, high FDG uptake in some benign lesions (eg, Hürthle cell adenoma or autonomous adenoma),[33] or low rate of true-positive results caused by inadequate cytologic examination, which could have obscured a malignant disease, particularly in the case of follicular lesions.

Thyroid FDG uptake also could be influenced by the state of thyroid function at the time of PET examination. In patients who have hypothyroidism, whole-body hypometabolism may result in slow clearance of FDG from the circulation. FDG is trapped intracellularly as FDG-6-phosphate and remains as such unless it is dephosphorylated by glucose-6-phosphatase. Hyperthyroidism has been shown to be associated with elevated glucose-6-phosphatase levels.[34] Hypothyroidism may conceivably result in a reduced glucose-6-phosphatase level in thyroid cells, which may prevent FDG-6-phosphate from being dephosphorylated and lead to increased FDG retention in the thyroid. It is also possible that augmented FDG uptake could be caused by a relatively high thyroid-stimulating hormone (TSH) level in patients who have hypothyroidism. In vitro studies have shown that TSH can significantly increase deoxyglucose uptake by the thyroid up to 700% in a dose-dependent manner.[35] TSH increases the expression of GLU1 and Glut4 in rat thyroid cells in time- and dose-dependent patterns.[36] The elevated TSH levels are also known to increase glucose metabolism by the thyroid cancer cells.[37] TSH stimulation increases the sensitivity of FDG-PET to detect thyroid carcinomas.[38,39] Thyroid FDG uptake depends on various factors, including the state of thyroid function, TSH levels, inflammation in the gland, and the presence of cancer cells. More studies at basic and clinical levels are needed to further determine factors that are most relevant to the uptake of FDG in normal tissue and in benign and malignant lesions.

BIOLOGIC BEHAVIOR OF THYROID CANCER INCIDENTALLY FOUND ON FLUORODEOXYGLUCOSE POSITRON EMISSION TOMOGRAPHY

Although the high cancer risk of incidental focal thyroid lesions warrants certain investigation, some factors, such as the extent of the known malignancy, comorbidities, and general clinical conditions, may not justify further evaluation in some patients. Knowledge of the biologic behavior of incidentally noted thyroid malignancy may be of importance in determining the extent to which the lesions should be investigated. Papillary carcinomas are the most common histologic type of cancer in the thyroid gland and usually have an indolent course. Based on experience gained over the past decade, most differentiated papillary cancers have low or no FDG uptake. It has been reported, however, that papillary carcinomas discovered by incidental FDG uptake show a high degree of malignancy with poor prognosis. Van den Bruel and colleagues[26] noted that of the three papillary thyroid carcinoma cases in their study, there was invasion of the thyroid capsule in two cells, which were associated with mediastinal lymph node metastasis containing undifferentiated tumor cells.

Are and colleagues[40] showed that in the 22 patients who had positive results on PET and a final diagnosis of primary thyroid malignancy, a greater number of patients (11/22, 50%) were noted to harbor tall-cell variant papillary thyroid carcinoma, which is substantially higher than the 4% to 8% rate in routinely detected thyroid cancers.[41,42] Patients with tall-cell variant papillary thyroid carcinoma cancer are known to have aggressive disease and poor prognosis compared with persons of the same age, sex, and size distribution who have papillary thyroid cancer.[43] Extrathyroid extension was noted in a high proportion of patients in the study (14 patients, 63%) and was much higher in patients with the tall-cell variant (10/11, 90%). Extrathyroid extension predicts a poor prognosis.[44] The authors concluded that thyroid malignancies incidentally detected on FDG-PET scan harbor a high rate of unfavorable prognostic features and may represent an aggressive variant of primary thyroid carcinoma, compared with malignancies in patients in the general population who do not have a history of cancer elsewhere in the body.

SUMMARY

In summary, any degree of FDG uptake in the thyroid gland on the PET scan is considered abnormal. Incidental FDG uptake in the thyroid, on the other hand, is not common, with a prevalence ranging from 2% to 3%, which is lower than that found with US. In patients with diffuse uptake, the probability of malignancy is low. Most such cases are caused by thyroiditis. Incidental focal FDG uptake in the thyroid harbors a 30% to 50% risk of malignancy, which is higher than noted with US. Most malignancies incidentally detected on FDG-PET are primary thyroid cancers, particularly papillary thyroid carcinoma, with unfavorable prognostic features. These malignancies may represent an aggressive variant of primary thyroid carcinoma, compared with those diagnosed in the general population. Thyroid metastasis from other malignancies is rare. Focal thyroid uptake should not be attributed to metastasis from the known primary malignancy in patients with proven cancer. The role of SUVs in distinguishing cancer from benign disease is controversial and unclear at this time.

REFERENCES

1. Ollenberger GP. Staging of lung cancer with integrated PET-CT. N Engl J Med 2004;350(1):86–7 [author reply: 86–7].
2. Terasawa T, Nihashi T, Hotta T, et al. 18F-FDG PET for posttherapy assessment of Hodgkin's disease and aggressive non-Hodgkin's lymphoma: a systematic review. J Nucl Med 2008;49(1):13–21.
3. Walker RC, Jones-Jackson LB, Martin W, et al. New imaging tools for the diagnosis of infection. Future Microbiol 2007;2(5):527–54.
4. Zhuang H, Duarte PS, Pourdehnad M, et al. The promising role of 18F-FDG PET in detecting infected lower limb prosthesis implants. J Nucl Med 2001; 42(1):44–8.
5. Nakamoto Y, Tatsumi M, Hammoud D, et al. Normal FDG distribution patterns in the head and neck: PET/CT evaluation. Radiology 2005;234(3):879–85.
6. Gordon BA, Flanagan FL, Dehdashti F. Whole-body positron emission tomography: normal variations, pitfalls, and technical considerations. AJR Am J Roentgenol 1997;169(6):1675–80.
7. Shreve PD, Anzai Y, Wahl RL. Pitfalls in oncologic diagnosis with FDG PET imaging: physiologic and benign variants. Radiographics 1999;19(1):150–1 [quiz: 61–77].
8. Tan GH, Gharib H. Thyroid incidentalomas: management approaches to nonpalpable nodules discovered incidentally on thyroid imaging. Ann Intern Med 1997;126(3):226–31.
9. Cohen MS, Arslan N, Dehdashti F, et al. Risk of malignancy in thyroid incidentalomas identified by fluorodeoxyglucose-positron emission tomography. Surgery 2001;130(6):941–6.

10. Kang KW, Kim SK, Kang HS, et al. Prevalence and risk of cancer of focal thyroid incidentaloma identified by 18F-fluorodeoxyglucose positron emission tomography for metastasis evaluation and cancer screening in healthy subjects. J Clin Endocrinol Metab 2003;88(9):4100–4.

11. Kim TY, Kim WB, Ryu JS, et al. 18F-fluorodeoxyglucose uptake in thyroid from positron emission tomogram (PET) for evaluation in cancer patients: high prevalence of malignancy in thyroid PET incidentaloma. Laryngoscope 2005;115(6):1074–8.

12. Are C, Hsu JF, Schoder H, et al. FDG-PET detected thyroid incidentalomas: need for further investigation? Ann Surg Oncol 2007;14(1):239–47.

13. Chen YK, Ding HJ, Chen KT, et al. Prevalence and risk of cancer of focal thyroid incidentaloma identified by 18F-fluorodeoxyglucose positron emission tomography for cancer screening in healthy subjects. Anticancer Res 2005;25(2B):1421–6.

14. Chu QD, Connor MS, Lilien DL, et al. Positron emission tomography (PET) positive thyroid incidentaloma: the risk of malignancy observed in a tertiary referral center. Am Surg 2006;72(3):272–5.

15. Bogsrud TV, Karantanis D, Nathan MA, et al. The value of quantifying 18F-FDG uptake in thyroid nodules found incidentally on whole-body PET-CT. Nucl Med Commun 2007;28(5):373–81.

16. Choi JY, Lee KS, Kim HJ, et al. Focal thyroid lesions incidentally identified by integrated 18F-FDG PET/CT: clinical significance and improved characterization. J Nucl Med 2006;47(4):609–15.

17. Yi JG, Marom EM, Munden RF, et al. Focal uptake of fluorodeoxyglucose by the thyroid in patients undergoing initial disease staging with combined PET/CT for non-small cell lung cancer. Radiology 2005;236(1):271–5.

18. Nam SY, Roh JL, Kim JS, et al. Focal uptake of (18)F-fluorodeoxyglucose by thyroid in patients with non-thyroidal head and neck cancers. Clin Endocrinol (Oxf) 2007;67(1):135–9.

19. King DL, Stack BC Jr, Spring PM, et al. Incidence of thyroid carcinoma in fluorodeoxyglucose positron emission tomography-positive thyroid incidentalomas. Otolaryngol Head Neck Surg 2007;137(3):400–4.

20. Yasuda S, Shohtsu A, Ide M, et al. Chronic thyroiditis: diffuse uptake of FDG at PET. Radiology 1998;207(3):775–8.

21. Karantanis D, Bogsrud TV, Wiseman GA, et al. Clinical significance of diffusely increased 18F-FDG uptake in the thyroid gland. J Nucl Med 2007;48(6):896–901.

22. Kurata S, Ishibashi M, Hiromatsu Y, et al. Diffuse and diffuse-plus-focal uptake in the thyroid gland identified by using FDG-PET: prevalence of thyroid cancer and Hashimoto's thyroiditis. Ann Nucl Med 2007;21(6):325–30.

23. Burguera B, Gharib H. Thyroid incidentalomas: prevalence, diagnosis, significance, and management. Endocrinol Metab Clin North Am 2000;29(1):187–203.

24. Boerner AR, Voth E, Theissen P, et al. Glucose metabolism of the thyroid in Graves' disease measured by F-18-fluoro-deoxyglucose positron emission tomography. Thyroid 1998;8(9):765–72.

25. Chen YK, Wang YF, Chiu JS. Diagnostic trinity: Graves' disease on F-18 FDG PET. Clin Nucl Med 2007;32(10):816–7.

26. Van den Bruel A, Maes A, De Potter T, et al. Clinical relevance of thyroid fluorodeoxyglucose-whole body positron emission tomography incidentaloma. J Clin Endocrinol Metab 2002;87(4):1517–20.

27. Davis PW, Perrier ND, Adler L, et al. Incidental thyroid carcinoma identified by positron emission tomography scanning obtained for metastatic evaluation. Am Surg 2001;67(6):582–4.

28. Nakhjavani MK, Gharib H, Goellner JR, et al. Metastasis to the thyroid gland: a report of 43 cases. Cancer 1997;79(3):574–8.

29. Lam KY, Lo CY. Metastatic tumors of the thyroid gland: a study of 79 cases in Chinese patients. Arch Pathol Lab Med 1998;122(1):37–41.

30. Dong C, Hemminki K. Second primary neoplasms among 53 159 haematolymphoproliferative malignancy patients in Sweden, 1958–1996: a search for common mechanisms. Br J Cancer 2001;85(7):997–1005.

31. Ueno M, Muto T, Oya M, et al. Multiple primary cancer: an experience at the Cancer Institute Hospital with special reference to colorectal cancer. Int J Clin Oncol 2003;8(3):162–7.

32. Ramos CD, Chisin R, Yeung HW, et al. Incidental focal thyroid uptake on FDG positron emission tomographic scans may represent a second primary tumor. Clin Nucl Med 2001;26(3):193–7.

33. Borner AR, Voth E, Wienhard K, et al. [F-18-FDG PET in autonomous goiter]. Nuklearmedizin 1999;38(1):1–6 [in German].

34. Karlander SG, Khan A, Wajngot A, et al. Glucose turnover in hyperthyroid patients with normal glucose tolerance. J Clin Endocrinol Metab 1989;68(4):780–6.

35. Filetti S, Damante G, Foti D. Thyrotropin stimulates glucose transport in cultured rat thyroid cells. Endocrinology 1987;120(6):2576–81.

36. Hosaka Y, Tawata M, Kurihara A, et al. The regulation of two distinct glucose transporter (GLUT1 and GLUT4) gene expressions in cultured rat thyroid cells by thyrotropin. Endocrinology 1992;131(1):159–65.

37. Moog F, Linke R, Manthey N, et al. Influence of thyroid-stimulating hormone levels on uptake of FDG in recurrent and metastatic differentiated thyroid carcinoma. J Nucl Med 2000;41(12):1989–95.

38. van Tol KM, Jager PL, Piers DA, et al. Better yield of (18)fluorodeoxyglucose-positron emission tomography in patients with metastatic differentiated thyroid carcinoma during thyrotropin stimulation. Thyroid 2002;12(5):381–7.

39. Chin BB, Patel P, Cohade C, et al. Recombinant human thyrotropin stimulation of fluoro-D-glucose positron emission tomography uptake in well-differentiated thyroid carcinoma. J Clin Endocrinol Metab 2004;89(1):91–5.

40. Are C, Hsu JF, Ghossein RA, et al. Histological aggressiveness of fluorodeoxyglucose positron-emission tomogram (FDG-PET)-detected incidental thyroid carcinomas. Ann Surg Oncol 2007;14(11): 3210–5.

41. Lam AK, Lo CY, Lam KS. Papillary carcinoma of thyroid: a 30-yr clinicopathological review of the histological variants. Endocr Pathol 2005;16(4):323–30.

42. Michels JJ, Jacques M, Henry-Amar M, et al. Prevalence and prognostic significance of tall cell variant of papillary thyroid carcinoma. Hum pathol 2007;38(2):212–9.

43. Prendiville S, Burman KD, Ringel MD, et al. Tall cell variant: an aggressive form of papillary thyroid carcinoma. Otolaryngol Head Neck Surg 2000; 122(3):352–7.

44. Siironen P, Louhimo J, Nordling S, et al. Prognostic factors in papillary thyroid cancer: an evaluation of 601 consecutive patients. Tumour Biol 2005;26(2): 57–64.

Adrenocortical Positron Emission Tomography/PET-CT Imaging

Rakesh Kumar, MD[a],*, Abass Alavi, MD, PhD[b], Stefano Fanti, MD[c]

KEYWORDS

- Adrenocortical imaging • FDG-PET
- ^{11}C-etomidate and ^{11}C-metomidate • Adrenal masses

The adrenal glands develop from the mesenchyme and play an important role in endocrine function. Maturation of adrenal medulla and cortex occurs within the first several years of life. The right adrenal gland has the shape of an elongated comma or an inverted letter V or Y and is located superior to the right kidney, medial to the right lobe of the liver, posterior to the inferior vena cava, and lateral to the crux of the right hemidiaphragm. The left adrenal gland has the shape of an inverted letter V, Y, or L and is located above and anterior to the upper pole of the left kidney, lateral to the descending aorta, and posterior to the body and tail of the pancreas. Because the right kidney is placed slightly below the level of the left kidney, both of the adrenal glands are seen at the same level in cross-sectional anatomy. The supero-inferior length of adrenals varies from 2 cm to 6 cm. The adrenal glands have two distinctly functioning portions: the outer cortex and the inner medulla. The adrenal medulla contains catecholamine- (epinephrine and non-epinephrine) producing cells, also known as chromaffin cells. The adrenal cortex is divided in to three zones and synthesizes three main hormones. The three zones are the zona glomerulosa, the zona fasciculata, and the zona reticularis, which produce aldosterone, cortisol and corticosterone, and dehydroepiadrosterone, respectively. All of these hormones are derived from cholesterol and share a common structural formula. With frequent use of computed tomography, the frequency of detecting adrenal masses is increasing. It has been estimated that as many as 10% to 20% of patients with essential hypertension may suffer from undiagnosed primary aldosteronism. Thus, the increased number of incidentally diagnosed adrenal masses, combined with underestimation of the prevalence of aldosteronism, lead to an increased demand for effective programs to characterize adrenal masses.

IMAGING MODALITIES

Various structural noninvasive imaging techniques, such as ultrasonography, CT, and MR imaging have been shown to be important in defining certain physiologic and pathologic characteristics of the adrenal glands, which are discussed in this article.

Computed Tomography

CT is the primary imaging modality for adrenal imaging. Widespread use of CT in clinical practice makes it an ideal noninvasive technique for evaluating adrenal gland morphology.[1] A variety of CT characteristics, such as lipid content, smooth border, maintenance of configuration, lack of calcification, and lack of enhancement after the contrast median is administered may allow for differentiation between adrenal adenomas and nonadenomas.[2–4] However, none of these characteristics are helpful in ruling out adrenal

a Department of Nuclear Medicine, All India Institute of Medical Sciences, New Delhi, India
b Department of Radiology, Hospital of the University of Pennsylvania, Philadelphia, PA, USA
c Department of Nuclear Medicine, S. Orsola-Malpighi Polyclinic, University of Bologna, Bologna, Italy
* Corresponding author.
E-mail address: rkphulia@yahoo.com (R. Kumar).

PET Clin 2 (2008) 331–339
doi:10.1016/j.cpet.2008.04.002

nonadenoma lesions with great accuracy.[5–7] To overcome these limitations, multiphase CT has been used, which demonstrates a higher level of accuracy. Adrenal masses with attenuation values less than 30 HU to 40 HU on 15-minute delayed contrast-enhanced CT (CECT) are almost always adrenal adenomas.[8] With multiphase CT, it is also possible to calculate the percentage of washout of the initial enhancement. The adrenal lesion is considered as benign if the relative washout value is greater than 40%.[3] However, the diagnosis of adrenal adenomas based on attenuation values and percentage wash out on multiphase CECT is often not feasible in routine clinical practice.

Magnetic Resonance Imaging

MR imaging is the second most commonly used imaging modality for characterization of indeterminate adrenal masses.[9–11] Because of high fluid content in malignant lesions of the adrenals, they appear bright on T2-weighted MR images. However, there is significant overlap on T1- and T2-weighted MR images of benign and malignant diseases. With the introduction of high field strength magnets (1.5T), chemical shift imaging and dynamic gadolinium-enhanced imaging, MR imaging has shown promising results in the characterization of adrenal gland lesions. Chemical shift MR imaging can distinguish adrenal adenoma from metastases. Schwartz and colleagues[12] studied 68 adrenal masses (23 malignant, 45 benign) in patients with known malignancy using echo-planar, fast spin-echo with and without fat suppression, and chemical shift pulse MR imaging sequences. The investigators demonstrated a sensitivity of 80% and specificity of 100%, with a cutoff adrenal mass-to-spleen ratio of 0.55. Chemical shift imaging primarily identifies protons in the body that are either located within water molecules or within lipid molecules, thus allowing separation of fat from water contributions in an image. The capability of chemical shift MR imaging plays an essential role in adrenal imaging because certain adrenal lesions contain a significant amount of lipids.

Functional Imaging

Adrenocortical lesions are heterogenous in nature and are characterized by the presence of secretary granules, the ability to produce biogenic amines, and the ability to produce polypeptide hormones. Therefore, the clinical behavior of these lesions is extremely variable; they can be functioning or inactive, slow-growing (well differentiated), or highly aggressive (poorly differentiated). Depending

on these features, different molecular imaging methods are used for their characterization.

Initially, molecular imaging was performed with analogs of cholesterol (^{131}I-19-iodocholestrol, ^{131}I-6β-iodomethyle-19-norcholestrol, and others), which act as a substrate for adrenal steroid hormone synthesis. After uptake, these analogs undergo esterification but are not further metabolized, and therefore serve as a marker of tissue cholesterol accumulation and the basis for adrenocortical imaging.[13,14] However, these radiopharmaceutics are not commonly used because of limited availability and suboptimal image quality. The results from these techniques are not available for at least 72 hours. In addition, the spatial resolution of gamma cameras with ^{131}I is greater than 1 cm to 2 cm, and therefore this technique tends to miss smaller lesions. Physiologic intestinal uptake of these radiopharmaceutics also makes interpretation of studies difficult.[14]

^{111}In-octreotide imaging exploits the overexpression of somatostatin receptors by adrenal tumors. It is helpful in detection of adrenal adenomas causing Cushing's syndrome.[15] Similar to other gamma camera-imaging modalities, ^{111}In-octreotide imaging cannot detect smaller lesions. Moreover, the results of these imaging techniques are available only 24 to 72 hours after the injection of the compound. In addition, the images are very difficult to interpret because of the complex biodistribution of this compound. Therefore, there is always a need for other noninvasive imaging techniques that can overcome the limitations of CT or MR imaging and gamma camera, which are based on the metabolic pathways that are associated with these lesions.

Molecular Imaging with Positron Emisson Tomography/Positron Emission Tomography-CT

18-F-fluorodeoxyglucose (FDG)-positron emission tomography (PET) is a new imaging modality that permits generation of important functional information about many disorders, and when combined with CT it reveals the exact location and the nature of the adrenal lesions. FDG is a glucose analog, which is taken up preferentially by malignant tissues because of increased glycolysis in neoplastic cells and release of hormones. Recently, many radiopharmaceutics have been developed for such approaches.^{18}F can be incorporated into a molecule, which in turn binds to receptors, undergoes metabolism by enzymes, or enters cells via transporters, such as ^{18}F-fluorodopamine and ^{18}F-fluorodihydroxyphenylalanine. Other positron-emitting radionuclides, such as ^{11}C, can be incorporated without changing the molecular structure or characteristics, such as ^{11}C-etomidate and ^{11}C-metomidate, among others.[16,17] Various PET radiopharmaceutics, which are being used and can be used in future for adrenocortical imaging, are listed in **Table 1**.

FDG is the most commonly used radiopharmaceutic for PET/PET-CT imaging.[18,19] Like glucose, FDG is transported into cells by means of a glucose transporter protein and begins to follow the glycolytic pathway. Once inside the cell, FDG is phosphorylated into ^{18}F-FDG-6-phosphate. However, ^{18}F-FDG-6-phosphate cannot continue through glycolysis because it is not a substrate for enzyme glucose-6-phosphate isomerase. As a result, ^{18}F-FDG-6-phosphate is biochemically trapped within the cell. This process of metabolic trapping constitutes the basis for FDG-PET imaging. Any pathology that demonstrates high glucose metabolism will be detected by the FDG-PET/PET-CT imaging. The degree of FDG uptake is often related to the grade of malignancy, and tumors that are characterized by rapid growth and aggressive histologic grading usually show high FDG uptake.

However, FDG-PET is not useful in all endocrine tumors because glucose metabolism is not much altered in these tumors. Rather, modern imaging techniques take advantage of the known metabolic activity of the endocrine tumor cells, such as uptake of hormone precursors, expression of certain receptors and transporters, and synthesis, storage, and release of hormones. Recently many radiopharmaceutics have been developed to take advantage of these well-characterized featured functions. For example, ^{18}F can be incorporated into a molecule that binds to receptors, undergoes metabolism by enzymes, or enters cells via transporters, such as ^{18}F-fluorodopamine and ^{18}F-fluorodihydroxyphenylalanine. Other positron-emitting radionuclides, such as ^{11}C, can be incorporated without changing the molecular structure or characteristics, for example ^{11}C-etomidate and ^{11}C-metomidate.[16,17] **Table 1** lists various PET radiopharmaceutics that are being used and can be used in the future for adrenocortical imaging.

The ^{11}C radiolabeled PET pharmaceutics, ^{11}C-etomidate and ^{11}C-metomidate, enter cells via transporters on the cell surface. ^{11}C-etomidate and ^{11}C-metomidate can be used to distinguish adrenocortical tumor from metastatic cancer based on targeting of specific enzymes expressed in adrenocortical tumors.[16,17] Both bind to 11β-hydroxylase, a key enzyme in cortisol and aldosterone synthesis. Both of these radiotracers offer specificity for identifying adrenocortical cells. All cortical lesions are easily identified because of

Table 1
Summary of radiopharmaceutics used for imaging of adrenocortical tumors

Radiopharmaceutic	Mechanism of Uptake	Isotope T1/2	Indication	Value
[18]-F-FDG	Glucose metabolism	120 min	Adrenocortical cancer, adrenal metastases	Good
[11]C-acetate	Glucose transport/ metabolic intermediate (tricarboxylic acid cycle intermediate)	20 min	Adrenocortical tumors	Possible
[11]C-etomidate	Adrenal cortical enzyme inhibitor	20 min	Adrenocortical tumors	Good
[11]C-metomidate	Adrenal cortical enzyme inhibitor	20 min	Adrenocortical tumors	Good
[18]F-fluoroethylester	Adrenal cortical enzyme inhibitor	120 min	Adrenocortical tumors	Possible

exceedingly high uptake of [^{11}C]-metomidate, whereas the noncortical lesions show very low uptake. Therefore, use of this radiopharmaceutic allows for differentiation of adrenocortical neoplasm from nonadrenocortical tumors with high sensitivity and specificity.[20]

However, these radiopharmaceutics cannot distinguish between benign and malignant adrenocortical lesions, such as benign adrenal neoplasm from adrenocortical carcinoma.[20,21] The other main limitation of ^{11}C-labeled radiopharmaceutics is the short half-life of 20 minutes, requiring an on-site cyclotron facility. In addition, these radiopharmaceutics need a sophisticated radio-synthesis facility. For these reasons, scans with these agents are mainly performed at research institutions as investigational studies.

CLINICAL APPLICATION
Adrenocortical Cancer

Most neuroendocrine tumors are well differentiated and are of low grade; FDG-PET has limited application in these tumors. However, FDG-PET/PET-CT plays an important role in diagnosis, staging, evaluating treatment response, and restaging of adrenocortical cancer and other malignant diseases, such as lymphoma, which are poorly differentiated and exhibit increased glucose metabolism.[22] FDG-PET imaging demonstrated more than 95% accuracy for distinguishing benign from malignant adrenocortical lesions, including secondary adrenocortical tumors (**Fig. 1**).[23–25]

Surgical excision remains the treatment of choice for patients with localized adrenocortical cancer. Conventional modalities have limitations and difficulties in differentiating postsurgical changes from recurrent disease. FDG plays a significant role in differentiation of postsurgical changes from recurrent adrenocortical cancer (**Fig. 2**). Distant metastases are noted in more than two-thirds of cases of adrenocortical cancer.[26] Therefore, early diagnosis and localization of metastatic disease is very important for further management of these patients. FDG-PET/PET-CT scanning can play an important role in detecting local recurrence and metastatic disease in patients with primary adrenocortical cancer.[26–28] Becherer and colleagues [27] prospectively studied 10 patients with adrenocortical cancer. The investigators demonstrated that FDG-PET imaging was 100% sensitive and 95% specific for this malignancy. They also observed that FDG-PET could detect multiple lesions that were not evident by other imaging modalities. Lebeulleux and colleagues[28] compared the use of PET/CT to conventional thoraco-abdominopelvic CT in the diagnosis of adrenocortical cancer. The investigators evaluated 269 lesions in 22 patients with adrenocortical cancer, and they noted the sensitivities for the detection of active lesions and the diagnosis of metastatic disease to be 90% and 93% for PET/CT and 88% and 82% for CT, respectively. Eighteen percent of the metastatic lesions were diagnosed with PET/CT only, and 7% with CT only. There were three false-positive lesions with PET/CT. Tumor size and mitotic rate were significantly associated with FDG uptake. High standardized uptake value (SUV) greater than 10 and the large volume of lesions with FDG uptake (>150 mL) were associated with poor survival. More recently, Mackie and colleagues[29] showed abnormal FDG uptake correctly indicated tumor recurrence in 10 out of 12 patients. One patient with no abnormal FDG activity had a morphologic abnormality subsequently proven to be a postoperative scar. Two patients, one with very small pulmonary lesions and one with a hepatic metastasis, had false-negative findings.

Hennings and colleagues[20] evaluated the role of ^{11}C-metomidate PET examinations in the management of adrenal tumors. They analyzed 75 histopathologic examinations from 73 patients: adrenocortical adenoma ($n = 26$), adrenocortical cancer ($n = 13$), adrenocortical hyperplasia ($n = 8$), pheochromocytoma ($n = 6$), metastasis ($n = 3$), and tumors of nonadrenal origin ($n = 19$). In this study, patients with pheochromocytomas, metastases to the adrenal gland, and nonadrenal masses were all ^{11}C-metomidate negative. SUV was higher in aldosterone-hypersecreting adenomas, and the SUV ratio between the tumor and the contralateral gland was significantly higher in all hormonally hypersecreting adenomas as well as in adrenocortical cancer. Khan and colleagues[21] studied ^{11}C-metomidate-PET in patients with adrenocortical cancer. In 11 patients, 13 PET findings were compared with those of CT and verified by histopathology. PET visualized all viable tumors with high tracer uptake, and revealed two additional lesions not seen on CT. Three tumors were not detected by PET and were confirmed to be necrotic by surgical and histopathologic examination. A true-negative observation was obtained by PET in the case of a suspected liver metastasis on CT.

Metastatic Disease to the Adrenals

FDG-PET/PET-CT has been found to play a definite role in the management of metastatic adrenal diseases (**Fig. 3**). The role of FDG-PET/PET-CT in differentiating benign and metastatic lesions in

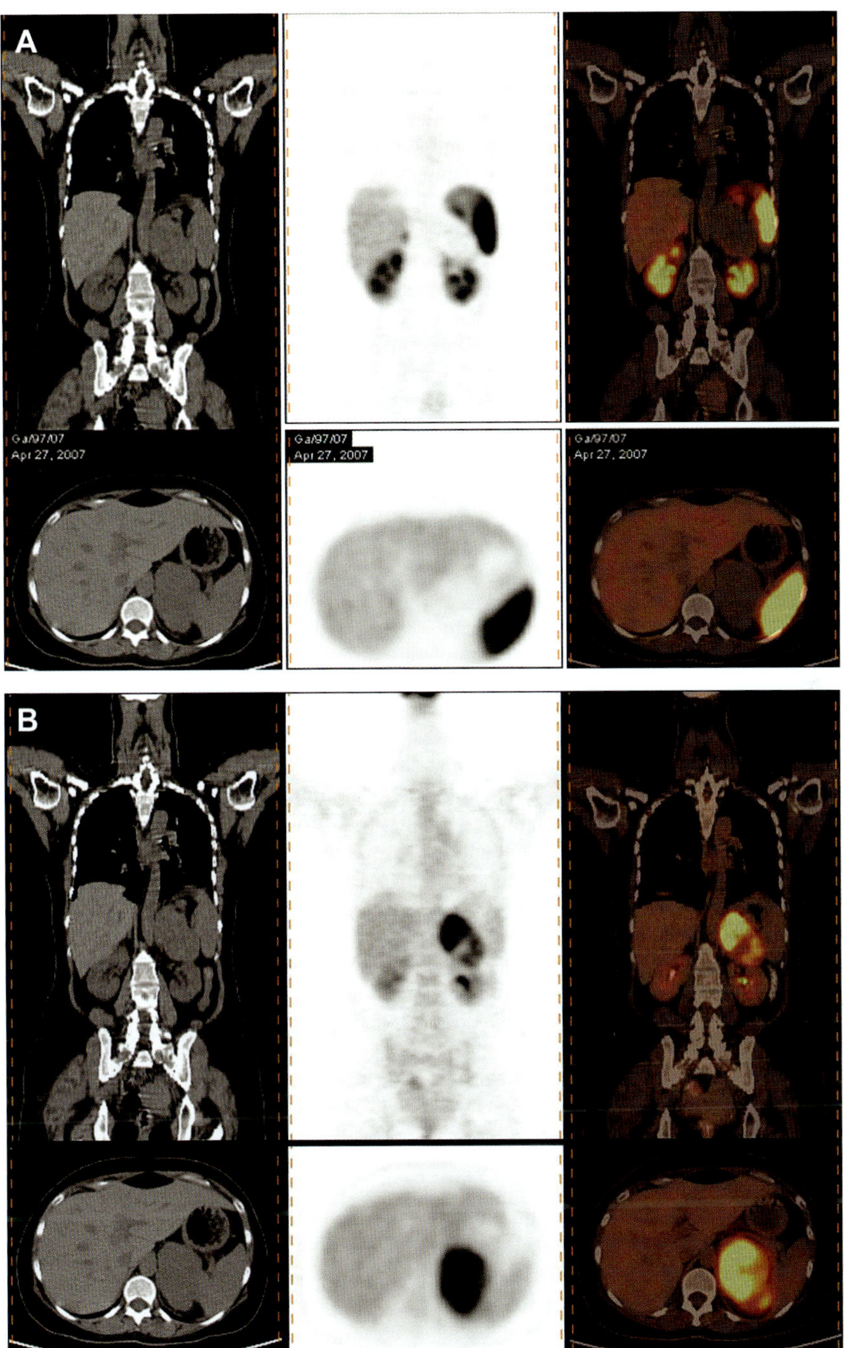

Fig. 1. A 45-year-old female presented with left adrenal mass seen on CT, underwent ^{68}Ga-DOTA-TOC PET-CT scan for further evaluation of adrenal mass. (*A*) Coronal and axial sections of CT, PET, and PET-CT demonstrated left adrenal mass with no radiotracer uptake. Patient underwent whole body ^{18}F-FDG PET-CT scan. (*B*) Coronal and axial sections of CT, PET and PET-CT demonstrated left adrenal mass with intense FDG uptake. These findings were suggestive of adrenocortical cancer. Biopsy done later confirmed the findings.

nonadrenal cancer patients has been evaluated by many investigators.[30–33] The results of all these studies are encouraging and justify the use of PET for metastatic disease evaluation in these patients, with a sensitivity and specificity ranging from 92% to 100% and from 80% to 100%, respectively. SUV values are often used as a predictor of malignancy, but the qualitative (visual)

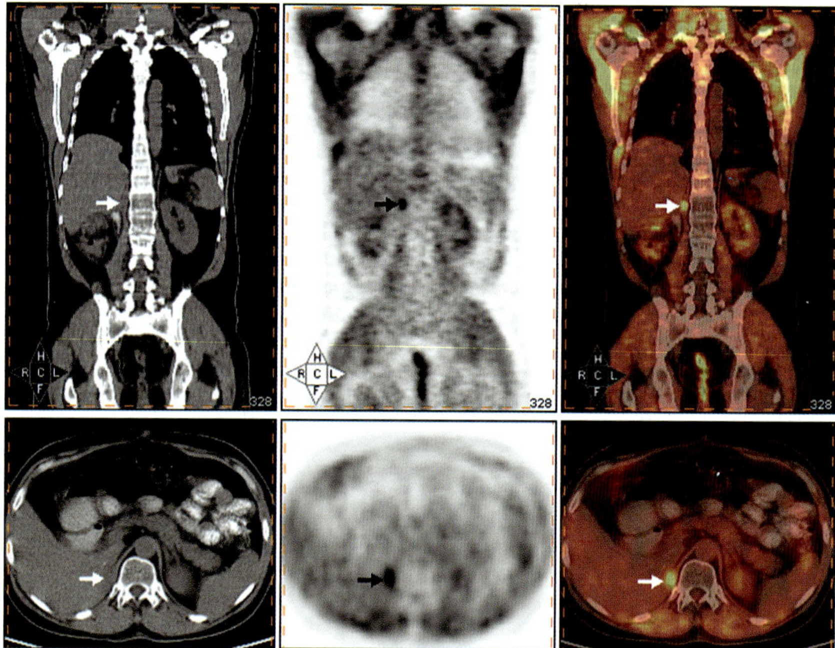

Fig. 2. A 43-year-old male, with a known case of right adrenocortical cancer, had right nephrectomy and adrenalectomy. A whole-body ^{18}F-FDG PET-CT scan was done to rule out any residual or recurrent disease. Coronal and axial sections of CT, PET and PET-CT demonstrated focus of abnormal FDG uptake in right adrenal bed (*arrows*). These findings were suggestive of recurrent adrenocortical cancer. Biopsy done later confirmed the findings.

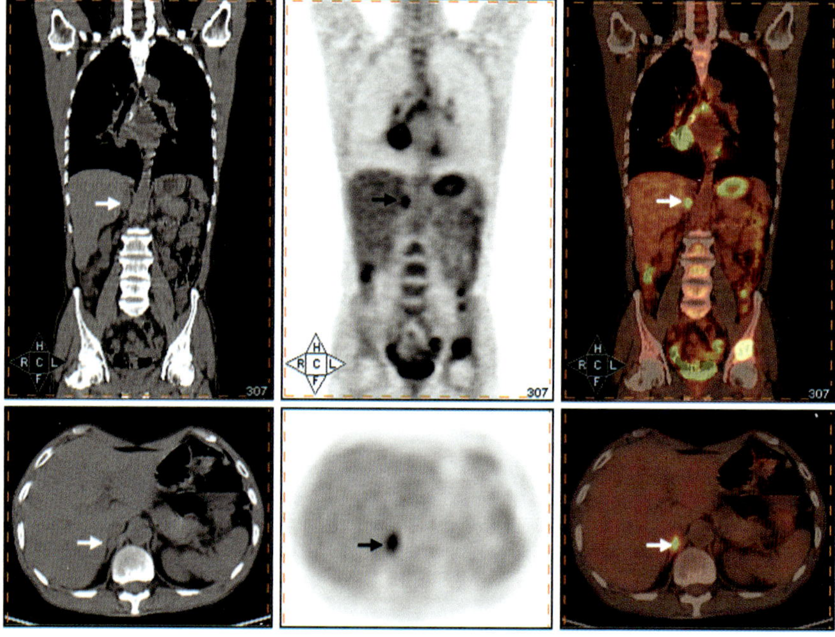

Fig. 3. A 65-year-old male presented with brain metastases of unknown primary. A whole-body [18] F-FDG PET-CT scan was done to find out the site of primary malignant pathology and other sites of metastses. Coronal and axial sections of CT, PET, and PET-CT demonstrated focus of abnormal FDG uptake in the right lung lower lobe, right adrenal bed, and multiple bones, including the left ilium. These findings were suggestive of primary cancer in the right lung with metastases in the right adrenal (*arrows*) and multiple bones.

examination comparing adrenal to liver uptake is quite effective and accurate.[32]

Some limitations of FDG-PET/PET-CT have been identified. FDG-PET cannot distinguish adrenocortical cancer from metastatic disease in the adrenal glands. Neither can it distinguish among pheochromocytoma, metastatic disease, and lymphoma, which generally exhibit high glycolytic activity. FDG-PET/PET-CT has also shown false-negative results in patients with very small lesions.[28,29]

Primary Aldosteronism

There is growing evidence that hyperaldosteronism contributes significantly to the development and severity of hypertension and its resistance to antihypertensive treatment. Plasma aldosterone levels have been shown to relate to blood pressure levels, especially in obese individuals. Hyperaldosteronism can be caused either by adrenal adenoma or by bilateral adrenal hyperplasia. The diagnosis of primary aldosteronism is commonly based on clinical and biochemical features. Although adrenal venous sampling is considered the standard of reference for determining the cause of primary aldosteronism, this method is technically demanding, costly, and time consuming. Noninvasive imaging modalities can play an important role in differentiating between the two main causes of primary aldosteronism: aldosterone-producing adenoma and bilateral adrenal hyperplasia. Imaging modalities such as CT, MR imaging, and adrenal scintigraphy, have also been used to determine the cause of primary aldosteronism. However, these conventional imaging modalities have lower sensitivity and specificity than PET imaging.[34] PET imaging with ^{11}C-metomidate has been shown to detect adrenal adenoma in patients with primary aldosteronism. ^{11}C-metomidate imaging clearly was able to distinguish cortical from noncortical adrenal masses (median SUVs of 18.6 and 1.9, respectively, P<.01).[23]

Hypercortisolism

[11]C-metomidate-PET has shown good results in depicting adrenocortical diseases in patients with hypercortisolism.[21,23,33] Patients with adenomas were found to have significantly higher tumor-to-normal adrenal ^{11}C-metomidate SUV ratios than did patients with non-adrenocortical tumors.[23] Most of the PET studies done with ^{11}C-metomidate clearly documented the fact that PET can differentiate adrenocortical lesions, such as cortical adenoma (nonsecreting and hypersecretory), cortical cancer, and macronodular

hyperplasia from non-adrenocortical tumors.[21,23,32,33] Hennings and colleagues[20] demonstrated sensitivity and specificity of 89% and 96%, respectively. The ^{11}C-metomidate uptake in hypersecreting adrenal adenomas and adrenocortical cancer is greater than in the contralateral normal cortex, suggesting contralateral suppression. ^{11}C-metomidate cannot differentiate benign hypercortisolism from malignant hypercortisolism. As noted above, FDG-PET/ PET-CT however, can easily distinguish these two conditions with high sensitivity and specificity.[26–28]

Incidentally Discovered Adrenal Lesions

The frequent and routine use of CT and MR imaging for evaluation of abdominal symptoms in non-cancer patients and metastatic disease in cancer patients is associated with a significant increase in the number of incidental findings. In the general population, 2% to 9% of patients are found to have benign adenomas.[35] Therefore, it is important to characterize adrenal masses accurately when they are discovered in cancer as well as non-cancer patients.

In a recent publication, ^{11}C-metomidate-PET was compared with CT and MR imaging in the characterization of adrenal incidental findings.[36] In 20 retrospectively and 24 prospectively evaluated adrenal incidental findings in patients who had undergone CT, MR imaging, and ^{11}C-metomidate-PET, the investigators demonstrated that CT and MR imaging combined can diagnose adrenocortical adenomas in most patients. In patients where CT and MR imaging have equivocal results, further characterization can be achieved by ^{11}C-metomidate-PET. In the authors' experience, there is no single imaging modality that can lead to a correct diagnosis. Rather, it is a battery of various imaging modalities that can lead to the proper management of adrenal incidental findings.

NEWER AGENTS

To overcome the limitation of the short half-life of ^{11}C, other PET radiopharmaceutics with a longer half-life are needed. 18 F- fluoroethylester (^{18}F-FETO) is a close analog of ^{11}C-etomidate and ^{11}C-metomidate. Similar to etomidate and metomidate, FETO is an inhibitor of 11β-hydroxylase enzyme, which plays an important role in the biosynthesis of cortisol and aldosterone, and has been shown to be a good target for adrenocortical lesions detected incidentally on CT scans. Wadsak and colleagues[37] evaluated the potency of ^{18}F-FETO as a PET tracer for the adrenal cortex in human beings. ^{18}F-FETO distribution was similar in all 10 scanned volunteers. Intense accumulation of ^{18}F-FETO was found in the adrenals, whereas moderate uptake was observed in some of the subjects' livers, renal calices, gallbladders, stomach walls, and pancreases. ^{18}F-FETO appears to be a valuable tracer for adrenocortical PET imaging, with the advantage of a longer half-life than C-11 (2 hours compared with 20 minutes) and with a high 11β-hydroxylase selectivity.

In conclusion, there is no single test that can characterize all adrenal masses. In most cases, CT and MR imaging combined can play an important role in characterization of adrenal masses. However, when the results of CT and MR imaging are equivocal, further characterization can be achieved using various functional imaging modalities. FDG-PET is particularly useful in detecting primary adrenocortical carcinoma or metastases from other primaries, but is usually not successful in detecting lower grade adrenal lesions, such as adenomas. The ^{11}C-labeled radiopharmaceutics—[11]C-etomidate and ^{11}C-metomidate—can distinguish between adrenal and nonadrenal lesions, because of their specificity, and may thus be useful in studying incidentally discovered adrenal masses.

REFERENCES

1. Gross MD, Korobkin M, Hussain H, et al. Adrenal gland imaging. In: Jameson JL, DeGroot LJ, editors. Endocrinology. 5th edition. Philadelphia: WB Saunders; 2005. p. 2425–53.

2. Hussain S, Belldegrun A, Seltzer SE, et al. Differentiation of malignant from benign adrenal masses: Predictive indices on computed topography. AJR Am J Roentgenol 1985;144:61–5.

3. Korobkin M. CT characterization of adrenal masses: the time has come. Radiology 2000;217:629–32.

4. Berland LL, Koslin DB, Kennedy PJ, et al. Differentiation between small benign and malignant adrenal masses with dynamic incremented CT. AJR Am J Roentgenol 1988;151:95–101.

5. Korobkin M, Brodeur FJ, Yutzy GG, et al. Differentiation of adrenal adenomas from non adenomas using CT attenuation values. AJR Am J Roentgenol 1996; 166:531–6.

6. Fishman EK, Deutch BM, Hartman DS, et al. Primary adrenocortical carcinoma: CT evaluation with clinical correlation. AJR Am J Roentgenol 1987;148:531–5.

7. Paivansalo M, Lahde S, Merikanto J, et al. Computed tomography in primary and secondary adrenal tumors. Acta Radiol 1988;29:519–22.

8. Korobkin M, Brodeur FJ, Francis IR, et al. CT time attenuation washout curves of adrenal adenomas and non adenomas. AJR Am J Roentgenol 1998; 170:747–52.

9. Mitchell DG, Crovello M, Matteucci T, et al. Benign adrenocortical masses: diagnosis with chemical shift MR imaging. Radiology 1992;185:345–51.

10. Outwater EK, Siegelman ES, Huang AB, et al. Adrenal masses: Correlation between CT attenuation value and chemical shift ratio at MR imaging with in-phase and opposed-phase sequences. Radiology 1996;200:749–52.

11. Haider MA, Ghai S, Jhaveri K, et al. Chemical shift MR imaging of hyper attenuating (>10 HU) adrenal masses: does it still have a role? Radiology 2004; 231:711–6.

12. Schwartz LH, Panicek DM, Koutcher JA, et al. Adrenal masses in patients with malignancy: prospective comparison of echo-planar, fast spin echo, and chemical shift MR imaging. Radiology 1995;197:421–5.

13. Gross MD, Shapiro B, Bouffard JA, et al. Distinguishing benign from malignant adrenal masses. Ann Intern Med 1988;109:613–8.

14. Gross MD, Avram A, Fig LM, et al. PET in the diagnostic evaluation of adrenal tumors. Q J Nucl Med Mol Imaging 2007;51:272–83.

15. Lumachi F, Zucchetta P, Marzola MC, et al. Usefulness of CT scan, MRI and radiocholesterol scintigraphy for adrenal imaging in Cushing's syndrome. Nucl Med Commun 2002;23:469–73.

16. Bergström M, Juhlin C, Bonasera TA, et al. PET imaging of adrenal cortical tumors with the 11-hydroxylase tracer 11C-metomidate. J Nucl Med 2000;41: 275–82.

17. Bergström M, Bonasera TA, Lu L, et al. In vitro and in vivo primate evaluation of carbon-11-etomidate and carbon-11-metomidate as potential tracers for PET imaging of the adrenal cortex and its tumors. J Nucl Med 1998;39:982–9.

18. Kumar R, Nadig M, Chauhan A. Positron emission tomography: clinical application in oncology: part I. Expert Rev Anticancer Ther 2005;5:1079–94.

19. Kumar R, Basu S, Anand V, et al. FDG-PET imaging for assessing inflammation and infection. Clin Microbiol Rev 2008;21:209–24.

20. Hennings J, Lindhe Ö, Bergström M, et al. [11C]metomidate positron emission tomography of adrenocortical tumors in correlation with histopathological findings. J Clin Endocrinol Metab 2006;91: 1410–4.

21. Khan TS, Sundin A, Juhlin C, et al. 11C-metomidate imaging of adrenocortical cancer. Eur J Nucl Med Mol Imaging 2003;30:403–10.

22. Kumar R, Xiu Y, Mavi A, et al. FDG-PET imaging in primary bilateral adrenal lymphoma: A case report and review of literature. Clin Nucl Med 2005;30:222–30.

23. Zettinig G, Mitterhauser M, Wadsak W, et al. Positron emission tomography imaging of adrenal masses: (18)F-fluorodeoxyglucose and the 11beta-hydroxylase tracer (11)C-metomidate. Eur J Nucl Med Mol Imaging 2004;31:1224–30.

24. Tenenbaum F, Groussin L, Foehrenbach H, et al. 18F-fluorodeoxyglucose positron emission tomography as a diagnostic tool for malignancy of adrenocortical tumours? Preliminary results in 13 consecutive patients. Eur J Endocrinol 2004;150:789–92.

25. Minn H, Salonen A, Friberg J, et al. Imaging of adrenal incidentalomas with PET using (11)C-metomidate and (18)F-FDG. J Nucl Med 2004;45:972–9.

26. Ng L, Libertino JM. Adrenocortical carcinoma: diagnosis, evaluation and treatment. J Urol 2003;169: 5–11.

27. Becherer A, Vierhapper H, Potzi C, et al. FDG-PET in adrenocortical carcinoma. Cancer Biother Radiopharm 2001;16:289–95.

28. Leboulleux S, Dromain C, Bonniaud G, et al. Diagnostic and prognostic value of 18-fluorodeoxyglucose positron emission tomography in adrenocortical carcinoma: a prospective comparison with computed tomography. J Clin Endocrinol Metab 2006;91:920–5.

29. Mackie G, Shulkin B, Ribeiro R, et al. Use of 18F]Fluorodeoxyglucose positron emission tomography in evaluating locally recurrent and metastatic adrenocortical carcinoma. J Clin Endocrinol Metab 2006;91:2665–71.

30. Blake MA, Slattery J, Kalra MK, et al. Adrenal lesions: characterisation with fused PET/CT image in patients with proved or suspected malignancy–initial experience. Radiology 2006;238:970–7.

31. Kumar R, Xiu Y, Yu JQ, et al. F18 -FDG PET in Evaluation of adrenal lesions in patients with lung cancer. J Nucl Med 2004;45:2058–62.

32. Jana S, Zhang T, Milstein DM, et al. FDG-PET and CT characterization of adrenal lesions in cancer patients. Eur J Nucl Med Mol Imaging 2006;33:29–35.

33. Kumar R, Anand V, Jana S. Adrenal Lesions: role of computed tomography, magnetic resonance imaging, 18fluorodeoxyglucose-positron emission tomography, and positron emission tomography/computed tomography. In: Hayat MA, editor. Instrumentation and Applications, Cancer Imaging, vol. 2. Philadelphia: Elsevier; 2008. p. 269–79.

34. Patel SM, Lingam RK, Beaconsfield TI, et al. Role of radiology in the management of primary aldosteronism. Radiographics 2007;27(4):1145–57.

35. Hedeland H, Ostberg G, Hokfelt B. On the prevalence of adrenocortical adenomas in an autopsy material in relation to hypertension and diabetes. Acta Med Scand 1968;184:211–4.

36. Hennings J, Hellman P, Ahlström H, et al. Computed tomography, magnetic resonance imaging and (11)C-metomidate positron emission tomography for evaluation of adrenal incidentalomas. Eur J Radiol 2007 Dec 13 [Epub ahead of print].

37. Wadsak W, Mitterhauser M, Rendl G, et al. [18F]FETO for adrenocortical PET imaging: a pilot study in healthy volunteers. Eur J Nucl Med Mol Imaging 2006;33:669–72.

PET Imaging of Pheochromocytoma

Sameer Khan, FRCR[a], Zarni Win, FRCR[a], Teresa Szyszko, FRCR[a],
Claire Lloyd, MRCP[a], Joel Dunn, MBBS[a], Abass Alavi, MD, PhD[b],
Adil AL-Nahhas, FRCP[a,*]

KEYWORDS

- Phaeochromocytoma • Paragangliomas
- Iodine-123-MIBG • ^{18}F-FDG • Gallium-68-DOTATATE

Pheochromocytomas (PCs) are tumors derived from chromaffin cells of the adrenal medulla that synthesize, store, metabolize, and usually, but not always, secrete catecholamines. Although PCs are the cause of hypertension in only a small number of patients, they can precipitate life-threatening hypertension or cardiac arrhythmias caused by excessive and episodic catecholamine secretion. The term "pheochromocytoma" (*phios* = dusky, *chroma* = color, and *cytoma* = tumor) refers to the color that the tumor cells acquire when stained with chromium salts. Tumors that arise from chromaffin cells outside the adrenal gland are termed extraadrenal PCs or paragangliomas.

More than 90% of PCs are located within the adrenal glands, and 98% occur within the abdomen. Extra-adrenal PCs may occur anywhere from the base of the skull to the floor of the pelvis. Common locations include the organ of Zuckerkandl and the retroperitoneum, bladder wall, and mediastinum. The prevalence of malignant PCs is approximately 10% (5%–26%), although higher rates have been reported in patients with extra-adrenal tumors,[1,2] with the most frequent sites of metastatic involvement being bone marrow, liver, and lung.

GENETICS AND CLINICAL BACKGROUND

Germ-line mutations in five different genes (autosomal dominant inheritance) have been identified as causes of PC and functional paragangliomas. The hereditary form of PC is associated with multiple endocrine neoplasia type 2a or 2B, neurofibromatosis type 1 (NF1), von Hippel Lindau syndrome, and familial functional paragangliomas and PCs caused by germ-line mutations of genes that encode succinate dehydrogenase (SDH) subunits B and D (SDHB and SDHD). It was previously thought that 10% of PCs were hereditary, but new studies demonstrate carriers of four different genes (von Hippel Lindau syndrome, RET protooncogene (RET), SDHB and SDHD) in up to 24% of patients.[3] Germ-line mutations of NF1, RET, SDH, and von Hippel Lindau syndrome genes allow sympathetic progenitors to escape from developmental apoptosis and subsequently lead to neoplastic transformation.[4] Likewise, mutations of SDHB and SDHD predispose their carriers to extra-adrenal and multifocal disease.[5]

PC occurs with equal frequency in men and women, typically in middle age but earlier in genetic syndromes. The prevalence in hypertensive patients is approximately 0.2% to 0.6%,[6,7] which increases to 4% to 5% in patients with incidentally discovered adrenal tumors.[8] PCs that present as incidental findings comprise up to 25% of all cases.[9] The clinical manifestations of PCs result from excessive secretion of norepinephrine, epinephrine, and rarely, dopamine. The most common signs include hypertension, tachycardia, palpitations, headache, sweating, and feelings of anxiety. Nausea, flushing, fever, and constipation also may occur. Stimulation of alpha-adrenergic receptors also results in glycogenolysis and gluconeogenesis, which can lead to diabetes mellitus. Sudden massive

[a] Departments of Nuclear Medicine and Imaging, Imperial College Healthcare Trust, Du Cane Road, London W12 0HS, United Kingdom
[b] Department of Radiology, Hospital of the University of Pennsylvania, 3400 Spruce Street, Philadelphia, PA 19104, USA
* Corresponding author. Department of Nuclear Medicine, Imperial College Healthcare Trust, Du Cane Road, London W12 0HS, United Kingdom
E-mail address: adil.al-nahhas@imperial.nhs.uk (A. AL-Nahhas).

PET Clin 2 (2008) 341–349
doi:10.1016/j.cpet.2008.04.003

catecholamine release can cause severe vasoconstriction, pulmonary edema, and fatal arrhythmias.

The diagnosis of PC by detection of catecholamines is practically difficult because catecholamines may be released intermittently or only at low rates. The metabolites of catecholamines, metanephrines, are constantly produced independently of catecholamine release and more accurately reflect tumor mass, however. Biochemical testing for PC should include measurement of plasma concentrations or urinary excretion of fractionated metanephrines. When these test results are positive, imaging studies are indicated.

IMAGING OF PHEOCHROMOCYTOMAS

PCs may be imaged with different modalities. CT and MR imaging provide structural information, and radiotracer-based studies reveal the molecular nature of the underlying disease processes. The latter can be divided into two categories, one bring specific for the catecholamine synthesis/secretion pathway, such as metaiodobenzylguanidine (MIBG), and the others that are nonspecific and include somatostatin receptor compounds (octreotide) and ^{18}F-fluorodeoxyglucose (FDG). Both types of agents can be imaged with either conventional scintigraphy or positron emission tomography (PET).

It is estimated that 98% of PCs are found within the abdomen; therefore, CT or MR imaging of the abdomen and pelvis is the initial modality for detecting the disease. CT is more readily available, is less expensive, and requires less time than MR imaging. Because of the relatively large radiation dose (approximately 10 mSv) associated with a CT scan of the abdomen and pelvis and relatively low contrast resolution for detecting abdominal lesions, MR imaging is the preferred modality, particularly in children and pregnant women. MR imaging is superior to CT for detecting extra-adrenal tumors, especially in the chest and neck.[10] Ultrasound and angiography are also useful in evaluating PC in the neck.[11] Detecting PCs in patients with the multiple endocrine neoplasia type 2 is easy because they are almost always intra-adrenal tumors. Anatomic imaging with CT and MR imaging is the first and often the only imaging modality used in most clinical settings. After anatomic imaging is performed and is diagnostic, molecular imaging techniques are of great value for monitoring response to therapy and determining the course of the disease.

CROSS-SECTIONAL IMAGING

On CT images, small PCs may appear with uniform attenuation, but in general, they are nonuniform with solid or cystic complex masses and contain calcification. Adrenal lesions with an average Hounsfield unit measurement of less than 10 on nonenhanced CT because of significant amounts of intracellular fat are usually accepted to be benign adenomas.[12]

After the administration of the contrast agents, PCs typically enhance avidly, although they may contain areas of nonenhancement caused by cystic structures. Assessing the washout profiles of adrenal lesions also can differentiate successfully the adenomas from malignant diseases. Adenomas have a relative washout rate more than 40% when delayed images are obtained 15 minutes after the administration of intravenous contrast agents. The washout rate in malignant lesions in general is less than 40%.[13] Unfortunately, PCs can demonstrate different and variable washout patterns, perhaps because of varied pathologic degeneration that produces abnormal capillary networks, which alter enhancement and washout with these agents.[13]

PCs typically demonstrate low signal on T1-weighted and high signal on T2-weighted images on MR imaging and enhance substantially after administration of gadolinium-based contrast agents.[14] As with CT, PCs may be incorrectly characterized as adenomas because of their variable contents. Approximately 65% of PCs are identified correctly, whereas the remaining 35% are classified incorrectly as malignant lesions or benign adenomas because of the atypical low signal intensity on T2-weighted MR images.[15] PCs cannot be excluded on the basis of a lack of high signal intensity on T2-weighted MR imaging. Cystic degeneration and hemorrhage within PCs can cause further diagnostic challenges on MR imaging.

SINGLE PHOTON IMAGING

Among single photon emitting radiopharmaceuticals, MIBG stands out as the most effective method for assessing patients with suspected PC. Developed by Wieland and colleagues,[16] the molecular structure of MIBG resembles that of norepinephrine, showing high affinity for the norepinephrine transporter system. It does not bind to adrenergic receptors, however, and is not metabolized within the catecholamine processing/secreting cells. Although MIBG was originally labeled with ^{131}I, this has been superseded by ^{123}I resulting in low radiation dose, superior image quality, and high sensitivity for detecting lesions.[17] The sensitivity of ^{123}I-MIBG in detecting PCs is 90% to 100% with a specificity of almost 100%.[18] Sensitivity for paragangliomas or malignant tumors is less impressive, however (71% and 56%, respectively).[19,20] Imaging is performed at 4 and 24 hours after administration of ^{123}I-MIBG using planar and single photon emission CT (SPECT) techniques.

Somatostatin receptor scintigraphy for assessing PC mainly deals with one compound, ^{111}In-DTPA-octreotide, because of expression of somatostatin receptor types 1, 2A, and 3 in these tumors. (Further details regarding somatostatin receptor scintigraphy are discussed in the section on PET imaging.) ^{111}In-DTPA-octreotide has been shown to be of limited value in the localization of PCs, however. In a study of patients with adrenal (n = 25) or metastatic PC (n = 8), the sensitivity rates of ^{111}In-DTPA-octreotide were 25% and 88%, respectively.[21]

POSITRON EMISSION TOMOGRAPHY

PET provides images with high spatial and contrast resolution, and improved image quality allows for detection of small lesions anywhere in the entire bodyThis technique in general delivers a lower radiation dose than modalities that use conventional radionuclides. Combined PET-CT (soon PET-MR imaging) imaging allows precise localization and definition of the abnormalities detected by both modalities.

The most commonly used radiopharmaceutical for this purpose is 2-[fluorine18] fluoro-2-de-oxy-D-glucose (FDG). FDG uptake reflects glycolysis in normal and pathologic states. It may be able to demonstrate disease activity in PC.[22] In addition to the metabolic imaging with FDG to examine patients who have PC, by targeting the noradrenergic transporter system by specific PET tracers, some specific molecular information can be gained with this technique. This includes the use of ^{18}F-fluorodopamine (^{18}F-DA), ^{18}F-dihydroxy phenylalanine (DOPA), ^{11}C-epinephrine, and ^{11}C-hydroxyephedrine (HED). An exciting new development uses somatostatin receptor (SSTR) imaging with ^{68}Ga-DOTA compounds for examining neuroendocrine tumors.

FLUORODEOXYGLUCOSE–POSITRON EMISSION TOMOGRAPHY IMAGING

FDG, a glucose analog, is the most widely used positron-emitting radiotracer in medical imaging. FDG is taken up by tumor and other cells with increased glycolytic activity, and once inside the cell, it undergoes phosphorylation by hexokinase to FDG 6-phosphate. The latter cannot be metabolized further and is trapped inside the cell because of low concentration of glucose-6-phosphatase in most tissues. Its uptake is nonspecific

and is seen in a variety of tumors and inflammatory and infectious processes.[22] Increased FDG uptake is demonstrated in PCs and adrenocortical carcinomas, but inactive adenomas and hypersecreting adenomas are not detected.[23]

Early reports have suggested that most PCs, whether benign or malignant, take up FDG. Shulkin and colleagues[22] identified PCs in 22 of 29 (76%) patients with the disease. Uptake was noted in a greater percentage of malignant (88%) than benign (58%) lesions, however, because of the high metabolic activity of neoplastic tumors. The overall sensitivity for localizing adrenal or metastatic phaeochromocytomas was reported to be 72%. The standardized uptake value did not distinguish benign from malignant lesions.[22] The same group found that some PCs with poor concentration of MIBG were well visualized with FDG and vice versa,[20] which is thought to be caused by the degree of cellular differentiation in these tumors. If a tumor contains dedifferentiated cells with loss of Glut 1 glucose transporter, it is probably malignant and takes up FDG.

Further confirmation of the use of FDG in detecting adrenal lesions came from Yun and colleagues,[24] who performed a retrospective analysis of scans of 50 patients with known or suspected malignancy and showed a sensitivity of 100% and specificity of 94%. This group used the liver as a reference point rather than background or blood pool activity for comparison with adrenal uptake of FDG. More recent publications also support the role of FDG-PET imaging in the assessment of PC and confirm its important role in the investigation of patients in whom ^{123}I-MIBG is negative.[25,26]

In general, FDG-PET imaging allows localization of PCs within and outside the adrenal glands, but it has poor specificity. In general, however, FDG-PET technique demonstrates more metastatic deposits than MIBG[22] in the body and is a useful imaging method when tumoral dedifferentiation has taken place.[20]

FUNCTIONAL POSITRON EMISSION TOMOGRAPHY IMAGING

[11]C- HED, a catecholamine analog, accumulates in organs with sympathetic innervation, including the heart, liver, kidney, pancreas, and spleen, with little or no uptake in the gastrointestinal tract. Because ^{11}C-HED uptake reflects catecholamine transport and storage, there is increased uptake in PCs and neuroblastomas. ^{11}C-HED has been shown to have a sensitivity of 90% to 92% and specificity of 100% for detecting PCs.[27,28] Imaging

with ^{11}C-HED is performed shortly after administering the tracer and continues up to 1 hour. Its short half-life (20 minutes) allows the administration of relatively high doses of the compound with an acceptable radiation dose. The short half-life of ^{11}C-HED is also a disadvantage, however, because it necessitates having an onsite cyclotron for making this agent.

Dopamine is an excellent substrate for the norephinephrine transporter 6-[18F]-fluorodopamine (^{18}F-DA), which is a positron-emitting analog of dopamine and a good substrate for the plasma membrane and intracellular vesicular transporters in catecholamine-synthesizing cells.[29] Several studies have suggested that ^{18}F-DA is a highly specific agent for localizing adrenal and extra-adrenal PCs, including metastatic lesions,[30–32] and has been found to be a superior tracer to MIBG.[20] It also has been used for imaging other tumors, such as neuroblastomas and ganglioneuromas.[33] There have been documented cases of aggressive PCs with widespread metastases in which there is no uptake with ^{18}F-DA but good uptake with FDG-PET. These are thought to be the dedifferentiated tumors.

[18]F-dihydroxyphenylalanine (^{18}F-DOPA), a precursor of dopamine, is used in brain imaging in patients who have Parkinson's disease but can be used in the imaging of neuroendocrine tumors, such as carcinoid, gastroenteropancreatic tumors, pediatric hyperinsulinism,[34–37] and PC. Its use is based on the capability of neuroendocrine tumors to take up, decarboxylate, and store amino acids such as DOPA. In a study reported by Hoegerle and colleagues,[38] all primary PCs and some extra-adrenal lesions in 14 patients were localized with a sensitivity and specificity of 100%. In this study, uptake was regarded as "massive" if it was comparable to that of the renal collecting system and "moderate" if distinctly weaker than the renal collecting system. In this study, PET and MR imaging provided the same sensitivity.[38]

An important feature of imaging with ^{18}F-DOPA is the lack of tracer uptake in normal adrenal glands; any uptake can be taken to be pathologic. This was observed not only in patients in this study but also in patients with suspected medullary thyroid cancer and gastrointestinal carcinoid.[39,40] It can differentiate scars from tumor recurrence and enables metabolic assessment of small structures, such as lymph nodes in metastasizing tumors.[38] The sensitivity of ^{18}F-DOPA can be improved with carbidopa, an inhibitor of dopa carboxylase. Timmers and colleagues[33] recently found that preadministration of carbidopa enhances the sensitivity of ^{18}F-DOPA-PET because additional lesions were detected in 3 of 11 patients.

SOMATOSTATIN RECEPTOR POSITRON EMISSION TOMOGRAPHY IMAGING

Somatostatin receptor imaging in PC provides a complementary alternative approach to single photon imaging with ^{123}I-labeled MIBG and metabolic imaging with FDG-PET. Somatostatin is a tetradecapeptide that contains 14 amino acids and is found throughout the central and peripheral nervous system and in various other tissues, such as the gasteroenteropancreatic tract, the kidneys, the adrenal and prostate glands, and immune cells. It primarily inhibits growth hormone release from the pituitary gland but has a wider role of acting as the inhibitor of the secretory and proliferative responses of target tissues [41] and inhibiting growth of normal and tumor tissues.[42]

Currently, five different somatostatin receptor subtypes (SSTR1–5) have been characterized and cloned.[43] These subtypes are encoded by five genes localized on separate chromosomes and belong to a family of seven transmembrane domain G protein-coupled receptors, which exhibit high binding affinity to the natural ligands SS-14 and SS-28. Somatostatin receptors are-expressed in many tissues, and multiple subtypes often coexist in the same cell. Some of these receptors are overexpressed in several human tumors, especially neuroendocrine tumors and their metastases.[44,45]

Data are limited on somatostatin receptor expression in PCs, which often express more than one somatostatin receptor, and it is still relatively unclear by which receptor subtype the functional responses of somatostatin analogs are mediated. It is generally accepted, however, that PCs express SSTR 3, 2A, and 5.[46–48] In a series of 52 PCs in 35 patients, Mundschenk and colleagues[48] showed that most tumors demonstrated positive staining for SSTR 3 (90%), with lower affinity for SSTR 2A (25%) and SSTR 5 (15%). More interestingly, there were different subcellular distributions of immunoreactive SSTR 3 among the SSTR 3-positive tumors, with most of the receptors distributed within the cytosol. Tumors larger than 1 cm, which possessed SSTR 2A, always could be detected with octreotide scintigraphy. When the SSTR 2A was absent, octreotide scintigraphy was only successful in the presence of membrane-associated SSTR 3 receptors. It is important to consider the cellular distribution of SSTR and the relative abundance of the different subtypes when considering and interpreting imaging with somatostatin analogs.

SOMATOSTATIN ANALOGS

SSTR-exhibiting tumors can be detected with conjugated somatostatin analogs such as ^{111}In-octreotide, which has been the mainstay of single photon somatostatin receptor scintigraphy for many years. Currently, several bifunctional chelators based on 1,4,7-triazacyclononane-N,N_,N_-triacetic acid and 1,4,7,10-tetraazacyclododecane-N,N_,N_,N_-tetraacetic acid (DOTA = 1,4,7,10-tetraazacyclodo-decane-1,4,7,10-tetraacetic acid) macrocycles are available for coupling to peptides and other biomolecules. [111In]DOTA-TOC and [90Y] DOTA-TOC have been shown to be effective in targeting and delivering therapeutic radiation doses to neuroendocrine tumors in animal models and patients.[48–51] Replacement of the alcohol group at the C-terminus of the octapeptide by a carboxylic acid group also led to increased SSTR 2 affinity.[52] Kwekkeboom and colleagues[53] showed higher tumor uptake with [177Lu-DOTA]-D-Phe[1]-Tyr[3]-Thr[8]-octreotide ([177Lu] DOTA-TATE) than [111]In [DOTA-Phe[1]-Tyr[3]] octreotide (DOTATOC) in six patients with somatostatin receptor-positive tumors. These new radiopeptides show distinctly higher SSTR 2 affinity compared with OctreoScan. They bind with high affinity only to SSTR 2, however, whereas their affinity to SSTR 5 is low and to that of SSTR 3 is almost negligible, and they have no affinity for SSTR 1 and SSTR 4.

A further study about the biologic activity profile of radiolabeled somatostatin analogs was undertaken by Wild and colleagues.[54] It resulted in a radiopeptide, [111In/90Y-DOTA]-1-Nal[3]-octreotide ([111In/90Y]DOTA-NOC), which had improved affinity to SSTR 2 and high affinity to SSTR 3 and SSTR 5 when compared with [111In/90Y]DOTA-TOC. Affinity toward SSTR 1 and 4 was low or absent. They found that ^{111}In-DOTA-NOC was superior to all somatostatin-based radiopeptides, which possess this particular type of binding profile, including DOTA-lanreotide. This preparation has three to four times higher binding affinity to SSTR 2 than ^{111}In/90YDOTA-Tyr3-octreotide (^{111}In/90Y-DOTATOC).

Even more recently, Ginj and colleagues[55,56] evaluated two new DOTA-based peptides, [111In-DOTA-Nal[3]-Thr[8]]-octreotide (DOTA-NOC-ATE) and [111In-DOTA-Bz-Thi[3]-Thr[8]]-octreotide (DOTA-BOC-ATE). The receptor affinity profile showed high affinity to SSTR 2, 3, and 5 and intermediate affinity to SSTR 4, whereas ^{111}In-DOTA-TOC showed affinity only to SSTR 2. Both radiopeptides internalized much more efficiently than ^{111}In-DOTATOC and the kidney uptake was significantly lower, which suggests great promise for potential clinical applications and targeted radiotherapy.

GALLIUM-68 DOTA COMPOUNDS

An appropriate somatostatin receptor compound can be synthesized with Gallium-68 (^{68}Ga), which is readily coupled to DOTA-peptides. [68]Ga is a positron emitter with a half-life of 68 minutes, and it decays mostly through emitting a positron with an energy of 1.92 MeV (maximum energy) and minimally through orbital electron capture. Its parent, germanium-68 ([68]Ge), is produced by an accelerator by using a Ga_2O_3 target. [68]Ge has a half-life of 270.8 days and decays by electron capture. [68]Ga positrons have a range of 8.1 mm in soft tissues, compared with a much smaller range of 2.4 mm for fluorine-18 positrons.

[68]Ga is available commercially as a [68]Ge/^{68}Ga generator. The [68]Ge-carrier column material is in the form of a TiO_2 matrix, maintaining it in the oxidative state (IV+). This arrangement has been shown to be especially stable minimizing [68]Ge breakthrough and contamination from the generator column material.[57,58] The [68]Ge/^{68}Ga generator comes in a form of a compact unit smaller than a [99]Mo/^{99m}Tc generator, thus requiring a small shelf space. Its long half-life allows its use for more than 1 year. The short half-life of the eluted ^{68}Ga permits suitable imaging for most applications while delivering an acceptable radiation dose to patients.

POSITRON EMISSION TOMOGRAPHY IMAGING WITH GALLIUM-68 DOTA PEPTIDES

Somatostatin receptor PET imaging of PCs can be achieved with ^{68}Ga DOTA peptides with great success. An important consideration before such imaging is undertaken is the location and the histopathologic differentiation of the tumor. As many as 20% of PCs are extra-adrenal in location[59] and tend to be malignant and frequently multicentric. The affinity of these extra-adrenal PCs to MIBG is lower when compared with adrenal PCs, and several authors have demonstrated that imaging with somatostatin analogs such as ^{111}In octreotide is more sensitive in the detection of malignant rather than benign PCs.[21,59–62] Further studies analyzing ^{123}I-MIBG–negative metastatic lesions have noted that imaging with somatostatin analogs is complementary to that of ^{123}I-MIBG scanning.[63–66] The exact reason for this observation is relatively unclear, but it has been postulated that the loss of MIBG affinity may be caused by

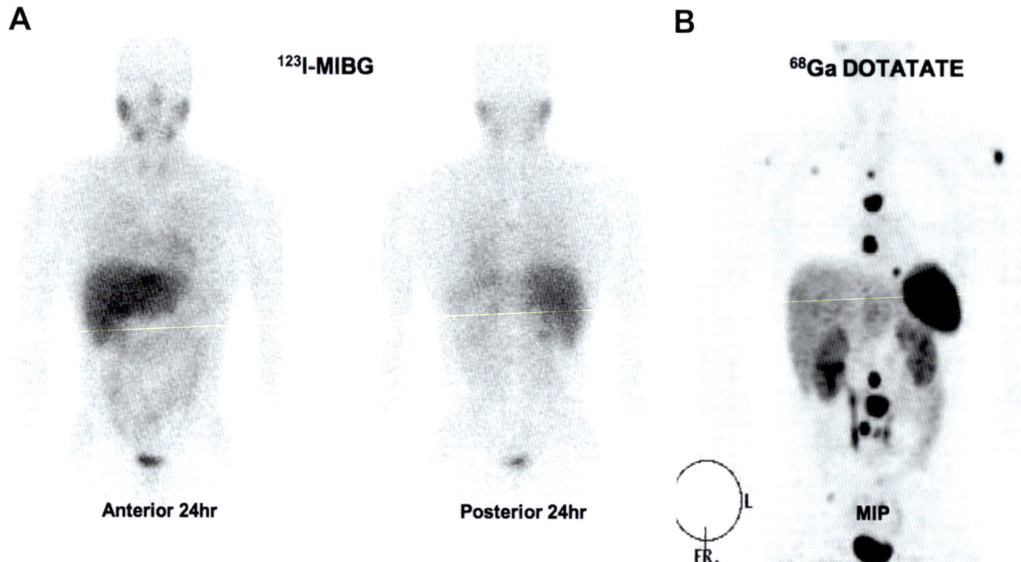

Fig. 1. Detection of metastatic PC in a 59-year-old man. Anterior and posterior whole-body ^{123}I-MIBG images obtained at 24 hours (*A*) show two lesions of minimally increased uptake in the mid-dorsal and lumbar spine. Maximum intensity projection (MIP) image of a ^{68}Ga DOTATATE PET study (*B*) shows high-grade uptake in a large number of bone metastases in thoracic and lumbar spine, ribs, and proximal humeral shafts. The ^{68}Ga DOTATATE PET image is clearly of higher resolution.

dedifferentiation of the tumor leading to the absence of catecholamine reuptake sites or abnormal storage granules that fail to concentrate catecholamines.[67]

The biodistribution of ^{68}Ga-DOTA-peptide PET is similar to that of ^{111}In octreotide, with uptake seen in the pituitary gland, liver, spleen, renal tract, bowel, and adrenal glands. It is usually not difficult to distinguish physiologic from pathologic uptake with fused anatomic information using PET/CT, especially of the suprarenal area. Imaging performed in patients with elevated biochemical markers increases the sensitivity of the examination.

Studies that describe the use of ^{68}Ga-DOTA-peptide PET in PCs are few at this time. In our small preliminary explanatory study of the viability of ^{68}Ga-DOTATATE PET imaging in PCs, we examined five patients who had previously undergone surgical resection of histologically proven malignant PCs and had clinical suspicion of recurrence. All underwent imaging with CT, ^{123}I-MIBG, and ^{68}Ga-DOTATATE PET.[68] Two patients (2/5) had negative results on [123]I -MIBG scintigraphy but had positive results on ^{68}Ga-DOTATATE PET. One patient (1/5) had weakly positive ^{123}I-MIBG scintigraphy but a strongly positive ^{68}Ga-DOTA-TATE PET. One patient (1/5) had positive results on ^{123}I-MIBG scintigraphy and positive results on ^{68}Ga-DOTATATE scans, but the latter detected an extra lesion. No lesions were detected in one patient (1/5) by any of the imaging modalities, including CT, but there was weakly positive uptake of ^{123}I-MIBG and ^{68}Ga-DOTATATE in a glomus jugulare tumor at the skull base, which was confirmed by MR imaging. The standardized uptake value (max) for the positive lesions ranged from 4.6 to 10.4, which indicated good tumor-to-background tracer uptake. We concluded that these findings provided a potential role for ^{68}Ga-DOTATATE PET in assessing malignant PCs, especially in those with no or little avidity for MIBG, as demonstrated by a recent case study (**Fig. 1**).[69]

Although there are limited data on the application of DOTA-peptide PET in PC, its role is well established in single photon somatostatin receptor scintigraphy with various agents, including ^{111}In octreotide. The introduction of somatostatin receptor PET agents to assess neuroendocrine tumors is an important evolution in medical imaging and should be validated for its optimal use in this setting.

SUMMARY

PCs and other neuroendocrine neoplasias are rare biochemically interesting tumors with unusual presentations and association with a variety of genetic syndromes. Malignant transformation is more common than previously thought, and developments in genetic screening and laboratory test have improved the detection rate in asymptomatic patients. Imaging is vital for diagnosis and follow-up after therapeutic interventions, and until recently, it has consisted of CT and MR imaging for structural characterization and ^{123}I-MIBG-PET for functional assessment. With novel PET radiopharmaceuticals, modern molecular imaging modalities have provided superior spatial and contrast resolutions and allowed for detection of the diseased sites with minimal discomfort to patients. One of the promising new radiopharmaceuticals is ^{68}Ga-DOTATATE, which has shown a higher sensitivity for detecting malignant lesions that express somatostatin receptors on cell membranes. We expect PET imaging to increasingly play a major role in the management of patients who have PC and other neuroendocrine tumors.

REFERENCES

1. Ahlman H. Malignant pheochromocytoma: state of the field with future projections. Ann N Y Acad Sci 2006;1073:449–64.
2. O'Riordain DS, Young WF Jr, Grant CS, et al. Clinical spectrum and outcome of functional extra-adrenal paraganglioma. World J Surg 1996;20(7):916–21.
3. Bornstein SR, Gimenez-Roqueplo AP. Genetic testing in pheochromocytoma: increasing importance for clinical decision making. Ann N Y Acad Sci 2006;1073:94–103.
4. Lee S, Nakamura E, Yang H, et al. Neuronal apoptosis linked to EglN3 prolyl hydroxylase and familial pheochromocytoma genes: developmental culling and cancer. Cancer Cell 2005;8(2):155–67.
5. Neumann HP, Pawlu C, Peczkowska M, et al. Distinct clinical features of paraganglioma syndromes associated with SDHB and SDHD gene mutations. JAMA 2004;292(8):943–51.
6. Ariton M, Juan CS, AvRuskin TW. Pheochromocytoma: clinical observations from a Brooklyn tertiary hospital. Endocr Pract 2000;6(3):249–52.
7. Omura M, Saito J, Yamaguchi K, et al. Prospective study on the prevalence of secondary hypertension among hypertensive patients visiting a general outpatient clinic in Japan. Hypertens Res 2004;27(3): 193–202.
8. Zelinka T, Eisenhofer G, Pacak K. Pheochromocytoma as a catecholamine producing tumor: implications for clinical practice. Stress 2007;10(2): 195–203.
9. Amar L, Servais A, Gimenez-Roqueplo AP, et al. Year of diagnosis, features at presentation, and risk of recurrence in patients with pheochromocytoma or secreting paraganglioma. J Clin Endocrinol Metab 2005;90(4):2110–6.
10. Sahdev A, Sohaib A, Monson JP, et al. CT and MR imaging of unusual locations of extra-adrenal paragangliomas (pheochromocytomas). Eur Radiol 2005;15(1):85–92.
11. Arslan H, Unal O, Kutluhan A, et al. Power Doppler scanning in the diagnosis of carotid body tumors. J Ultrasound Med 2000;19(6):367–70.
12. Boland GW, Lee MJ, Gazelle GS, et al. Characterization of adrenal masses using unenhanced CT: an analysis of the CT literature. AJR Am J Roentgenol 1998;171(1):201–4.
13. Caoili EM, Korobkin M, Francis IR, et al. Adrenal masses: characterization with combined unenhanced and delayed enhanced CT. Radiology 2002;222(3):629–33.
14. Blake MA, Kalra MK, Maher MM, et al. Pheochromocytoma: an imaging chameleon. Radiographics 2004;24(Suppl 1):S87–99.
15. Varghese JC, Hahn PF, Papanicolaou N, et al. MR differentiation of phaeochromocytoma from other adrenal lesions based on qualitative analysis of T2 relaxation times. Clin Radiol 1997;52(8):603–6.
16. Wieland DM, Wu J, Brown LE, et al. Radiolabeled adrenergi neuron-blocking agents: adrenomedullary imaging with [131I]iodobenzylguanidine. J Nucl Med 1980;21(4):349–53.
17. Lynn MD, Shapiro B, Sisson JC, et al. Portrayal of pheochromocytoma and normal human adrenal medulla by m-[123I]iodobenzylguanidine: concise communication. J Nucl Med 1984;25(4):436–40.
18. Zapanti E, Ilias I. Pheochromocytoma: physiopathologic implications and diagnostic evaluation. Ann N Y Acad Sci 2006;1088:346–60.
19. Erickson D, Kudva YC, Ebersold MJ, et al. Benign paragangliomas: clinical presentation and treatment outcomes in 236 patients. J Clin Endocrinol Metab 2001;86(11):5210–6.
20. Ilias I, Yu J, Carrasquillo JA, et al. Superiority of 6-[18F]-fluorodopamine positron emission tomography versus [131I]-metaiodobenzylguanidine scintigraphy in the localization of metastatic pheochromocytoma. J Clin Endocrinol Metab 2003; 88(9):4083–7.
21. van der Harst E, de Herder WW, Bruining HA, et al. [(123)I]metaiodobenzylguanidine and [(111)In]octreotide uptake in begnign and malignant pheochromocytomas. J Clin Endocrinol Metab 2001;86(2): 685–93.
22. Shulkin B, Thompson N, Shapiro B, et al. Phaeochromocytomas: imaging with 2-[fluorine-18]fluoro-2-deoxy-D-glucose PET. Radiology 1999;212:35–41.
23. Avram A, Fig L, Gross M. Adrenal gland scintigraphy. Semin Nucl Med 2006;36:212–27.
24. Yun M, Kim W, Alnafisi N, et al. 18F-FDG PET in characterizing adrenal lesions detected on CT or MRI. J Nucl Med 2001;42:1795–9.
25. Mackenzie IS, Gurnell M, Balan KK, et al. The use of 18-fluorodeoxyglucose positron emission tomography scanning in the assessment of metaiodobenzylguanidine negative phaeochromocytoma. Eur J Endocrinol 2007;157(4):533–7.

26. Chrisoulidou A, Kaltsas G, Ilias I, et al. The diagnosis and management of malignant phaeochromocytoma and paraganglioma. Endocr Relat Cancer 2007;14(3):569–85.

27. Shulkin B. PET scanning with hydroxyephedrine: an approach to the localisation of phaeochromocytoma. J Nucl Med 1992;33:1125–31.

28. Trampal C, Engler H, Juhlin C, et al. Phaeochromocytomas: detection with 11C hydroxyephedrine PET. Radiology 2004;230:423–8.

29. Eisenhofer G. The role of neuronal and extraneuronal plasma membrane transporters in the inactivation of peripheral catecholamines. Pharmacol Ther 2002;91:35–62.

30. Pacak K, Linehan W, Eisenhofer G, et al. Recent advances in genetics, diagnosis, localization and treatment of phaeochromocytoma. Ann Intern Med 2001;134:315–29.

31. Pacak K, Goldstein D, Doppman J, et al. A "pheo" lurks: novel approaches for locating occult pheochromocytoma. J Clin Endocrinol Metab 2001;86: 3641–6.

32. Pacak K, Eisenhofer G, Carrasquillo J, et al. 6-18F fluorodopamine positron emission tomographic (PET) scanning for diagnostic localisation of phaeochromocytoma. Hypertension 2001;38:6–8.

33. Timmers H, Hadi M, Carrasquillo J, et al. The effects of carbidopa on uptake of 6-18F-fluoro-L-DOPA in PET of pheochromocytoma and extra-adrenal abdominal paraganglioma. J Nucl Med 2007; 48(10):1599–606.

34. Becherer A, Szabo M, Karanikas G, et al. Imaging of advanced neuroendocrine tumors with 18F-FDOPA-PET. J Nucl Med 2004;45(7):1161–7.

35. Koopmans KP, de Vries EG, Kema IP, et al. Staging of carcinoid tumors with 18F-DOPA PET: a prospective, diagnostic accuracy study. Lancet Oncol 2006; 7(9):728–34.

36. Ambrosini V, Tomassetti P, Rubello D, et al. Role of 18F-DOPA PET/CT imaging in the management of patients with 111 In-pentetreotide negative GEP tumors. Nucl Med Commun 2007;28(6):473–7.

37. Hardy OT, Hernandez-Pampaloni M, Saffer JR, et al. Diagnosis and localization of focal congenital hyperinsulinism by 18F-fluorodopa PET scan. J Pediatr 2007;150(2):140–5.

38. Hoegerle S, Nitzsche E, Altehoefer C, et al. Pheochromocytomas: detection with 18F DOPA whole-body PET initial results. Radiology 2002;222:507–12.

39. Hoegerle S, Altehoefer C, Ghanem N, et al. Whole body 18F DOPA PET for detection of gastrointestinal carcinoid tumors. Radiology 2001;220:373–80.

40. Hoegerle S, Altehoefer C, Ghanem N, et al. 18F DOPA positron emission tomography for tumor detection in patients with medullary thyroid carcinoma and elevated calcitonin levels. Eur J Nucl Med 2001;28:64–71.

41. Patel YC. General aspects of the biology and function of somatostatin. In: Weil C, Muller EE, Thorner MO, editors. Basic and clinical aspects of neuroscience. Berlin: Springer-Verlag; 1992. p. 1–16.

42. Weckbecker G, Raulf F, Stolz B, et al. Somatostatin analogs for diagnosis and treatment of cancer. Pharmacol Ther 1993;60:245–64.

43. Patel YC. Somatostatin and its receptor family. Front Neuroendocrinol 1999;20(3):157–98.

44. Reubi JC, Waser B. Concomitant expression of several peptide receptors in neuroendocrine tumors: molecular basis for in vivo multireceptor tumor targeting. Eur J Nucl Med Mol Imaging 2003;30(5): 781–93.

45. Reubi JC, Waser B, Schaer JC, et al. Somatostatin receptor sst1-sst5 expression in normal and neoplastic human tissues using receptor autoradiography with subtype-selective ligands. Eur J Nucl Med 2001;28:836–46.

46. Hofland LJ, Liu Q, Van Koetsveld PM, et al. Immunohistochemical detection of somatostatin receptor subtypes sst1 and sst2A in human somatostatin receptor positive tumors. J Clin Endocrinol Metab 1999;84:775–80.

47. Reubi JC, Waser B, Khosla S, et al. In vitro and in vivo detection of somatostatin receptors in pheochromocytomas and paragangliomas. J Clin Endocrinol Metab 1992;74:1082–9.

48. Mundschenk J, Unger N, Schulz S, et al. Somatostatin receptor subtypes in human pheochromocytoma: subcellular expression pattern and functional relevance for octreotide scintigraphy. J Clin Endocrinol Metab 2003;88:5150–7.

49. de Jong M, Bakker WH, Krenning EP, et al. Yttrium-90 and indium-111 labelling, receptor binding and biodistribution of [DOTA0,D-Phe1,Tyr3] octreotide: a promising somatostatin analogue for radionuclide therapy. Eur J Nucl Med 1997;24:368–71.

50. Otte A, Herrmann R, Heppeler A, et al. Yttrium-90-DOTATOC: first clinical results. Eur J Nucl Med 1999;26:1439–47.

51. Otte A, Mueller-Brand J, Dellas S, et al. Yttrium-90-labelled somatostatin-analogue for cancer treatment. Lancet 1998;351:417–8.

52. Reubi J, Schaer J, Waser B, et al. Affinity profiles for human somatostatin receptor subtypes SST1–SST5 of somatostatin radiotracers selected for scintigraphic and radiotherapeutic use. Eur J Nucl Med 2000;27:273–82.

53. Kwekkeboom DJ, Bakker WH, Kooij PP, et al. [177Lu-DOTA0,Tyr3] octreotate: comparison with [111In-DTPA0] octreotide in patients. Eur J Nucl Med 2001;28:1319–25.

54. Wild D, Schmitt JS, Ginj M, et al. DOTA-NOC, a high-affinity ligand of somatostatin receptor subtypes 2, 3 and 5 for labelling with various radiometals. Eur J Nucl Med Mol Imaging 2003;30(10):1338–47.

55. Ginj M, Chen J, Walter MA, et al. Preclinical evaluation of new and highly potent analogues of octreotide for predictive imaging and targeted radiotherapy. Clin Cancer Res 2005;11(3):1136–45.

56. Ginj M, Schmitt JS, Waser B, et al. Design, synthesis, and biological evaluation of somatostatin-based radiopeptides. Chem Biol 2006;13(10):1081–90.

57. McElvany KD, Hopkins KT, Welch MJ. Comparison of 68Ge/68Ga generator systems for radiopharmaceutical production. Int J Appl Radiat Isot 1984;35:521–4.

58. Meyer GJ, Maecke H, Schuhmacher J, et al. 68Ga-labelled DOTA-derivatised peptide ligands. Eur J Nucl Med Mol Imaging 2004;31:1097–104.

59. Whalen RK, Althausen AF, Daniels GH. Extra-adrenal pheochromocytoma. J Urol 1992;147:1–10.

60. Jalil ND, Pattou FN, Combemale F, et al. Effectiveness and limits of pre-operative imaging studies for the localisation of pheochromocytomas and paragangliomas: a review of 282 cases. Eur J Surg 1998;164:23–8.

61. Mozley PD, Kim CK, Moshin J, et al. The efficacy of iodine-123-MIBG as a screening test for pheochromocytoma. J Nucl Med 1994;35:1138–44.

62. Maurea S, Lastoria S, Caraco C, et al. The role of radiolabeled somatostatin analogs in adrenal imaging. Nucl Med Biol 1996;23:677–80.

63. Steinert H, Lehnert H, Bockisch A, et al. Detection of malignant pheochromocytoma tumor sites by 111-In-octreotide scintigraphy. Eur J Nucl Med 1993; 20:843.

64. Hoefnagel CA. MIBG and radiolabeled octreotide in neuroendocrine tumors. Q J Nucl Med 1995;39: 137–9.

65. Lastoria S, Maurea S, Vergara E, et al. Comparison of labeled MIBG and somatostatin analogs in imaging neuroendocrine tumors. Q J Nucl Med 1995;39: 145–9.

66. Tenenbaum F, Lumbroso J, Schlumberger M, et al. Comparison of radiolabeled octreotide and meta-iodobenzylguanidine (MIBG) scintigraphy in malignant pheochromocytoma. J Nucl Med 1995;36:1–6.

67. Shulkin BL, Koeppe RA, Francis IR, et al. Phaeochromocytomas that do not accumulate metaiodobenzylguanadine: localization with PET and administration of FDG. Radiology 1993;186:711–5.

68. Win Z, Al-Nahhas A, Towey D, et al. 68Ga-DOTATATE PET in neuroectodermal tumors: first experience. Nucl Med Commun 2007;28(5):359–63.

69. Win Z, Rahman L, Murrell J, et al. The possible role of 68Ga-DOTATATE PET in malignant abdominal paraganglioma. Eur J Nucl Med Mol Imaging 2006; 33(4):506.

PET/CT in Neuroendocrine Tumors: Evaluation of Receptor Status and Metabolism

Vikas Prasad, MD[a], Valentina Ambrosini, MD, PhD[b],
Abass Alavi, MD, PhD[c], Stefano Fanti, MD[b],
Richard P. Baum, MD, PhD[a],*

KEYWORDS

- Neuroendocrine tumors • PET/CT
- Somatostatin receptor imaging • Ga-68 • F-18 DOPA

Neuroendocrine tumors (NETs) include a diverse group of neoplasms characterized by their endocrine function and specific histologic characteristics. Previously known as carcinoid tumors, the term coined by Oberndorfer[1] in 1907 for small intestinal lesions, most NET neoplasms were wrongly thought to originate from the neural crest. Recently, the origin of these tumors has been traced to pluripotent stem cells or differentiated neuroendocrine cells.[2] APUD-oma (amine precursor uptake and decarboxylation), gastroenteropancreatic (GEP) tumor, islet cell tumor, neuroendocrine carcinoma, and other names have been suggested to cover the wide variety of tumor types that belong to the NET group.[2]

The most common sites from which NETs originate are the bronchus/lungs and GEP tract and, less often, the skin, adrenal glands, thyroid, and genital tract.[3] NETs that have a common origin from the foregut, midgut, or hindgut share similar functional manifestations, histochemistry, and secretory granules.[3] Histologically, NETs can be classified based on the degree of differentiation

(**Box 1**).[4,5] A new tumor, node, and metastasis staging scheme has been proposed for foregut NETs, and it has been shown by some groups to have good correlation with prognosis. The presence or absence of symptoms because of biogenic amines and hormones has been the basis for classifying NETs as functional or nonfunctional tumors. Nearly 33% to 50% of all NETs are nonfunctional, whereas the rest are associated with various symptoms.

Numerous factors are known to have an influence on survival and prognosis of patients, among which the presence of liver metastases is the single most important factor. A correlation has been found between the size of the primary tumor and the probability of metastases for small intestinal carcinoids. Metastases to the liver can be found in 15% to 25% of tumors if the tumor diameter is in less than 1 cm, 58% to 80% if it is 1 to 2 cm, and more than 75% if the tumor size is more than 2 cm.[3] These prognostic factors make it essential to use reliable diagnostic indicators before treating patients with a particular treatment regimen.

[a] Department of Nuclear Medicine and Center for PET/CT, Zentralklinik Bad Berka GmbH, Robert Koch Allee-9, 99437 Bad Berka, Germany

[b] Department of Nuclear Medicine, University of Bologna, Policlinico S. Orsola-Malpighi, via Massarenti 9, 40138 Bologna, Italy

[c] Department of Radiology, Hospital of the University of Pennsylvania, 3400 Spruce Street, 110 Donner Building, Philadelphia, PA 19104, USA

* Corresponding author.
E-mail address: info@rpbaum.de (R.P. Baum).

PET Clin 2 (2008) 351–375
doi:10.1016/j.cpet.2008.04.007

> **Box 1**
> **World Health Organization classification of endocrine tumors**
>
> - Well-differentiated endocrine tumor
> - Well-differentiated endocrine carcinoma
> - Poorly differentiated endocrine carcinoma
> - Mixed exocrine-endocrine tumor
> - Tumor-like lesion

DIAGNOSIS OF NEUROENDOCRINE TUMORS: HISTOPATHOLOGY, BIOCHEMICAL INVESTIGATION, STRUCTURAL IMAGING

Biochemical Investigations

The most validated markers for the diagnosis and the follow-up of carcinoid tumors include[2]

1. Chromogranin A (CGA)
2. 5-Hydroxyindoleacetic acid (urinary metabolite of serotonin)
3. Gastrin
4. Serotonin
5. Pancreastatin
6. Neurokinin A (substance K)

For follow-up, serial measurements of these markers are made every 3 to 6 months. The absolute value of CGA is not a determinate of tumor burden; nor can it rule out or confirm metastases. Changes in CGA level by 25% over the baseline are considered significant. There has been a concordance between the CGA levels and the findings on ^{131}I-metaiodobenzylguanidine (MIBG) scintigraphy. A CGA level in the reference range has been found to be highly predictive of normal scintigraphy results. Several other conditions lead to elevated levels of CGA, however, such as hypergastrinemia caused by electrochromaffin-like cell hyperplasia secondary to proton pump inhibitors, renal insufficiency, and severe hypertension. Circadian rhythm of CGA warrants the need for blood sampling at approximately the same time at every visit for follow-up purposes.

In cases in which gastrinoma is suspected (history of abdominal pain, diarrhea, and gastroesophageal reflux disease) a fasting gastrin level should be measured. For insulinoma, an elevated insulin level should be demonstrated in fasting state. C-peptide and serum glucose levels are also measured. For pheochromocytoma, metanephrines, catecholamines, and their metabolites should be measured in the blood and urine.[2,3]

Histopathology

In the past, NETs were lumped together as a single entity because they were characterized by their propensity to stain with silver and have abnormal levels of neuroendocrine tissue markers, such as chromogranin, neuron-specific enolase, and synaptophysin, when immunohistochemical methods were used. The recent World Health Organization classification and the new tumor, node, and metastasis staging[6] scheme have taken into consideration the different histopathologic behavior of these tumors in characterizing them further. These classifications have been shown to have good correlation with prognosis.

Structural Diagnostic Imaging

Surgical resection remains the mainstay of treatment of NET; after biochemical confirmation, the next step in the diagnostic algorithm is to stage the disease. Although CT and MR imaging are accurate in providing correct anatomic location of the lesions, structural imaging methodologies are of limited use in diagnosing an unknown tumor and defining its prognosis of NETs. The extent of the tumor, in terms of metastases, often can be underestimated based on morphologic criteria because molecular changes precede structural alterations with most disorders. Likewise, in therapy monitoring, the size criteria are often inadequate for detecting early response. The role of ultrasound (US) in the diagnosis of NET is also limited and depends largely on the site of disease. For the detection of liver metastases, US has a high diagnostic accuracy. In cases in which a gastric or pancreatic primary tumor is suspected, endoscopic US is of diagnostic value.

Molecular/Metabolic Imaging

Positron emission tomography (PET) is increasingly being used for detecting disease at the molecular/metabolic level. The feasibility of fusing functional imaging (PET or single photon emission CT [SPECT]) with structural imaging (CT/MR imaging) overcomes certain shortcomings of purely functional imaging alone for diagnostic and therapeutic purposes. This article covers only the role of PET and PET/CT in the management of patients with NETs. It includes potential PET radiopharmaceuticals used for this purpose, imaging protocols, and the various indications for PET or PET/CT in NETs.

POSITRON EMISSION TOMOGRAPHY RADIOPHARMACEUTICALS

PET radiopharmaceuticals can be directed toward assessing receptor expression or characterizing

Table 1
Positron emission tomography radiopharmaceuticals for the diagnosis of neuroendocrine tumors

	Radiopharmaceutical	Receptor/Metabolic Target	Indication and Comments
PET	^{18}F-FDG	Glycolytic pathway	All NETs. Sensitivity in NET is low compared with other radiopharmaceuticals. Useful for undifferentiated NET. Observation of flip-flop mechanism with SMS-R PET
	^{68}Ga-DOTA-NOC	Somatostatin receptor (pansomatostatin, high affinity for SSTR2, 3, and 5)	All SSTR + VE NETs
	^{68}Ga-DOTA-TOC	Somatostatin receptor (highest affinity for SSTR2)	All SSTR + VE NETs
	^{11}C-5-HTP	Serotonin production pathway	All serotonin-producing NETs
	^{11}C-DOPA	Dopamine production pathway	Pheochromocytoma, paraganglioma, neuroblastoma. Short half-life, cost of production, and difficulty in obtaining ^{11}C-labeled compounds pose limitations for this compound
	^{18}F-DOPA	Dopamine production pathway	Pheochromocytoma, paraganglioma, neuroblastoma, glomus tumor
	^{18}F-FDA	Catecholamine precursor	Pheochromocytoma, paraganglioma, neuroblastoma
	^{64}Cu-TETA-octretoide	Somatostatin receptor	All SSTR + VE NETs
	^{18}F-FP-Gluc-TOCA	Somatostatin receptor	All SSTR + VE NETs
	^{11}C-ephedrine	Catecholamine transporter	Pheochromocytoma, neuroblastoma, study of sympathetic nervous system
	^{11}C-hydroxyephidrine	Catecholamine transporter	Pheochromocytoma, neuroblastoma, study of sympathetic nervous system

Abbreviation: VE; positive.

the intratumoral metabolic processes. The metabolic events and receptor targets that are currently being examined by PET are as follows (**Table 1**):

Receptor targets:
1. Somatostatin receptor expression
2. Miscellaneous other peptide receptors

Metabolic processes:
1. Serotonin production pathway
2. Biogenic amine storage
3. Catecholamine transport
4. Glucose metabolism

Receptor-Targeting Radiopharmaceuticals

Somatostatin receptor-based radiopharmaceuticals

The abundance of somatostatin receptor (SSTR) expression on NETs (**Table 2**) has resulted in the development of several radiopharmaceuticals that are directed toward these sites. Among the five different SSTR types, most NETs express SSTR2, with a low percentage expressing SSTR1 and SSTR5.[7–9]

The currently used somatostatin radiopharmaceuticals (**Table 3**) are derivatives of octreotide, lanreotide, or vapreotide and show variable binding to SSTR.[8,10–12] ^{68}Ga-DOTA-TOC was the first radiopharmaceutical used for PET imaging of NETs. Wild and colleagues[11,12] have shown that the compound ^{68}Ga-DOTA-NOC has three to four times higher binding affinity to SSTR2, 3, and 5 than ^{68}Ga-DOTA-TOC, which results in detection of a wide range of SSTR-positive tumors (pansomatostatin analog) and has a significant effect on diagnosis, staging, and therapy of NETs and various other somatostatin-receptor expressing tumors. Other somatostatin analogs, such as DOTA-NOC-ATE [(DOTA-1Nal^3, Thr8)-octreotide] and DOTA-BOC-ATE [(DOTA, BzThi^3, Thr^8)-octreotide], are in the preclinical stages of development. SSTR antagonists, (NH(2)-CO-c(DCys-Phe-Tyr-DAgl(8)Me,2-naphthoyl)-Lys-Thr-Phe-Cys)-OH (sst(3)-ODN-8) and (sst(2)-ANT), also have been labeled with ^{111}In. They have been shown to be superior to SSTR agonists (in mice model) for in vivo targeting of SSTR2- and SSTR3-rich tumors.[13,14]

^{68}Ga is eluted from a ^{68}Ga/68Ge generator. Currently, several vendors supply Ga-68/Ge-68 generators, making it widely accessible around the globe. ^{68}Ga (t$_{1/2}$ = 68 min) is a positron emitter with an 89% positron emission rate and a negligible gamma emission (1077 keV) of only 3.2%. The long half-life of the mother radionuclide ^{68}Ge (270.8 days) makes it possible to use the generator for approximately 9 to 12 months, depending on the requirement.

Table 2
Somatostatin receptor expression on different tumors

Tumor Types	Receptor Subtypes
Gastroenteropancreatic NET	SSTR1, SSTR2, SSTR5
Neuroblastoma	SSTR2
Meningioma	SSTR2
Breast carcinoma	SSTR2
Medulloblastoma	SSTR2
Lymphoma	SSTR2, SSTR5
Renal cell carcinoma	SSTR2
Paraganglioma	SSTR1, SSTR2, SSTR3
Small-cell lung cancer	SSTR2
Hepatoma	SSTR2
Prostate carcinoma	SSTR1
Sarcoma	SSTR1, SSTR2, SSTR4
Inactive pituitary adenoma	SSTR1, SSTR2, SSTR3, SSTR5
Growth hormone–producing pituitary adenoma	SSTR2, SSTR3, SSTR5
Gastric carcinomas	SSTR1, SSTR2, SSTR5
Ependydomas	SSTR1
Pheochromocytoma	SSTR1, SSTR2, SSTR5

Table 3
Affinity profiles (IC$_{50}$) of somatostatin receptor subtypes for different somatostatin analogs used in diagnostic imaging with positron emission tomography/CT or single photon emission CT

Somatostatin Analogs	SSTR1	SSTR2	SSTR3	SSTR4	SSTR5
Native somatostatin (S28)	5.2	2.7	7.7	5.6	4.0
In-DTPA-octreotide	> 10,000	22	182	> 1000	237
In-DOTA-[Tyr3]octreotide (DOTA-TOC)	> 10,000	4.6	120	230	130
DOTA-lanreotide (DOTA-LAN)	> 10,000	26	771	> 10,000	73
DOTA-[Tyr3]octreotate (DOTA-TATE)	> 10,000	1.5	> 1000	453	547
Y-DOTA-TOC	> 10,000	11	389	> 10,000	114
Ga-DOTA-TOC	> 10,000	2.5	613	> 1000	73
In-DOTA[1-Nal3]octreotide (DOTA-NOC)	> 10,000	2.9	8	227	11.2
Y-DOTA[1-Nal3]octreotide (DOTA-NOC)	> 1000	3.3	26	> 1000	10.4
In-DOTA-NOC-ATE	> 10,000	2	13	160	4.3
In-DOTA-BOC-ATE	> 1000	1.4	5.5	135	3.9

IC50 is expressed in nanomoles (lower value represent higher receptor affinity).

For labeling purposes, the ^{68}Ga eluate is first concentrated and purified using a micro chromatography method as described by Rösch and colleagues.[15,16] After preconcentration and purification of the initial generator eluates, [68]Ga(III) is re-eluted with 400 μL 98% acetone/0.05 N HCl solution (2×10^{-5} mol HCl). This fraction is used for labeling of DOTA-octreotide derivatives, such as DOTA-TOC, DOTA-NOC, or DOTA-TATE. For the production of ^{68}Ga-DOTA-NOC, 1 GBq ^{68}Ga is put into a vial containing 30 to 50 μg of the peptide. Subsequently, ^{68}Ga-DOTA-NOC is purified and finally eluted using 0.5 mL ethanol into 4.5 mL of isotonic saline. Radiolabeling yields of more than 95% can usually be achieved within 15 minutes. Overall, 370 to 700 MBq of ^{68}Ga-DOTA-NOC are obtained within 20 minutes.

For DOTA-TOC, the processed eluate containing [68]Ga (up to 700 MBq) is added to 4 to 4.5 mL pure H_2O in the reagent vial containing 7 to 14 nmol DOTA-TOC with addition of HERPES buffer. ^{68}Ga-labeled DOTA-derived octreotides are purified from unreacted ^{68}Ga species by reversed phase chromatography. The reaction mixture is then passed through a small C18 cartridge; after washing the cartridge with 5 mL H_2O, the ^{68}Ga-labeled peptide is recovered with 200 to 400 μL of pure ethanol. A radiolabeling yield of 88% at approximately 99°C is achieved within 10 minutes with specific activities of up to 450 MBq/μmol of peptide.[17]

Miscellaneous peptides

Several other peptides have been developed by radiopharmacists for imaging NETs. Bombesin labeled with ^{68}Ga is one such peptide that is being investigated in undifferentiated prostate cancers, breast carcinomas, small-cell lung cancer, and renal cell carcinomas and some NETs. VIP, a 28 amino acid peptide that was initially isolated from porcine intestine, has been studied for imaging of neuroendocrine GEP tumors, especially VIPomas.[18–22] Other peptides that have been used for receptor scintigraphy of NETs include cholecystokinin (CCK-B), gastrin, minigastrin and others. Work is ongoing to determine the best peptide for targeting these tumors.[23–28]

Table 4
Drugs that interfere with vesicular monoamine transporters, leading to wrong interpretation of ^{123}I/^{131}I-MIBG single photon emission CT, ^{11}C-E/^{11}C-HED/^{18}F-FDA positron emission tomography scans

Mechanism	Drugs
Uptake-1 inhibition	Sympathomimetics (eg, cocaine, opioids)
	Tricyclic antidepressants (eg, amitryptaline, imipramine, ioxapine)
	Antipsychotic/antiemetics (eg, phenithiazines, thioxanthenes, butyrophenones)
	Antihypertensive/cardiovascular agents
	Tetracyclic antidepressants (eg, Maprotiline, mirtazapine)
Inhibition of granular uptake	Antihypertensive/cardiovascular agents (eg, Reserpine)
	For movement disorders (eg, tetrabenazine)
Competitive inhibition of granular uptake	Sympathomimetic (eg, norepinephrine)
	Antidepressants (eg, serotonin)
	Antihypertensives (eg, guanethidine)
Depletion of storage granules	Antihypertensive/cardiovascular agents (eg, Reserpine, guanethidine, labetolol, bethanidine)
	Sympathomemtics (eg, phenylephrine, phenylpropanolamine, ephedrine, pseudoephedrine, amphetamine, dobutamine, dopamine, metarminol)
Increased uptake and retention	Antihypertensives/calcium channel blockers (eg, angiotensin-converting enzyme inhibitors)

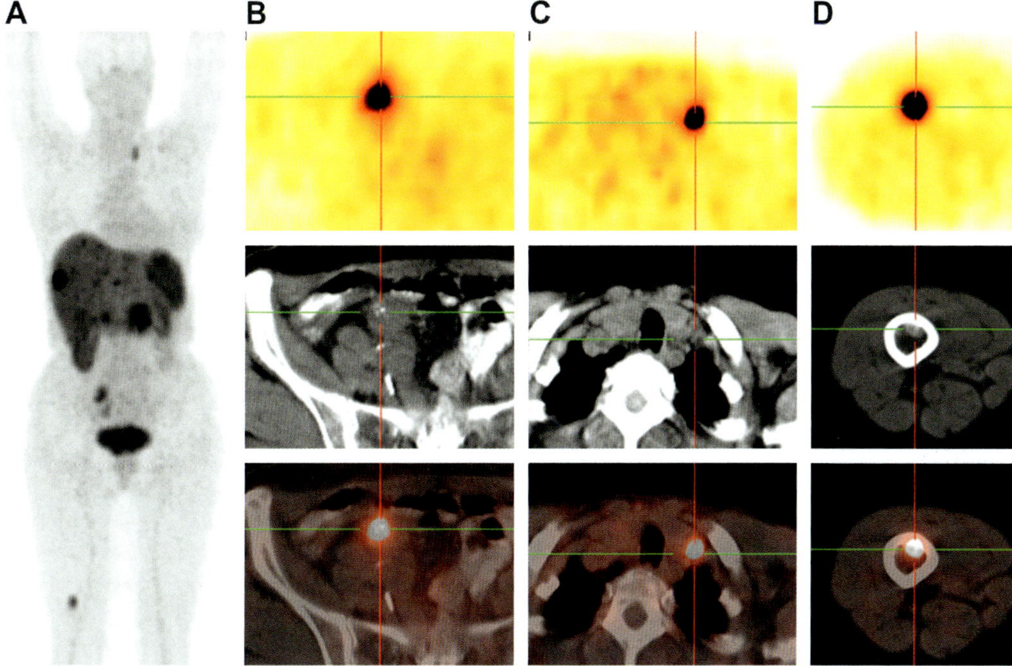

Fig. 1. Ga-68 DOTA-TATE PET/CT: Whole-body diagnosis ("one stop shop"). Maximum intensity projection image (*A*) showing an abdominal lesion, liver metastases, a left supraclaviular lesion and a hot spot in the right thigh. Transversal PET/CT slices reveal the primary tumor (previously unknown) in the ileum (*B*), a left parathyroidal lymph node metastasis (*C*) and a bone marrow metastasis (also previously unknown) in the right distal femur (*D*).

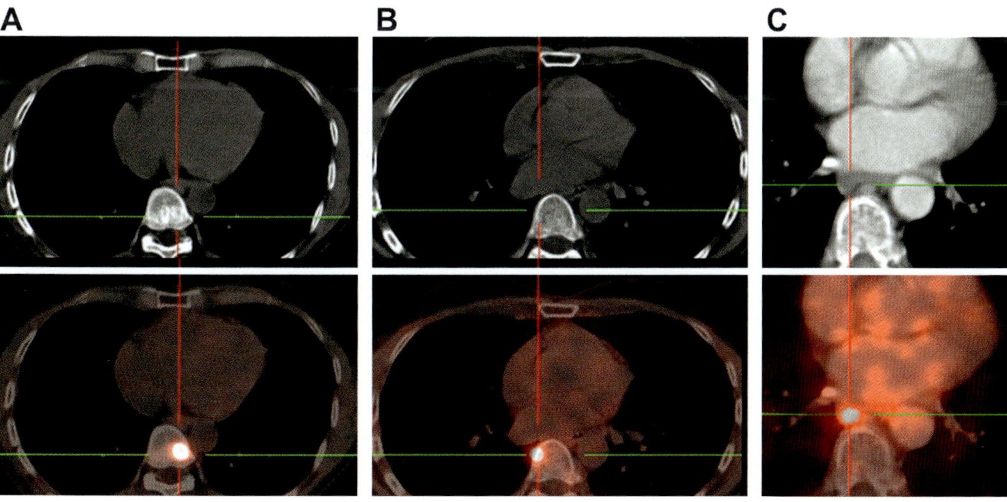

Fig. 2. Ga-68 DOTA-NOC PET/CT: Accuracy and sensitivity of disease localization. Osteoblastic metastases in thoracic vertebra (*A*), bone marrow metastasis (*B*) without anatomical alteration on CT (in MRI size 3 mm in diameter), and small prevertebral/paracardiac metastasis of neuroendocrine tumor (*C*).

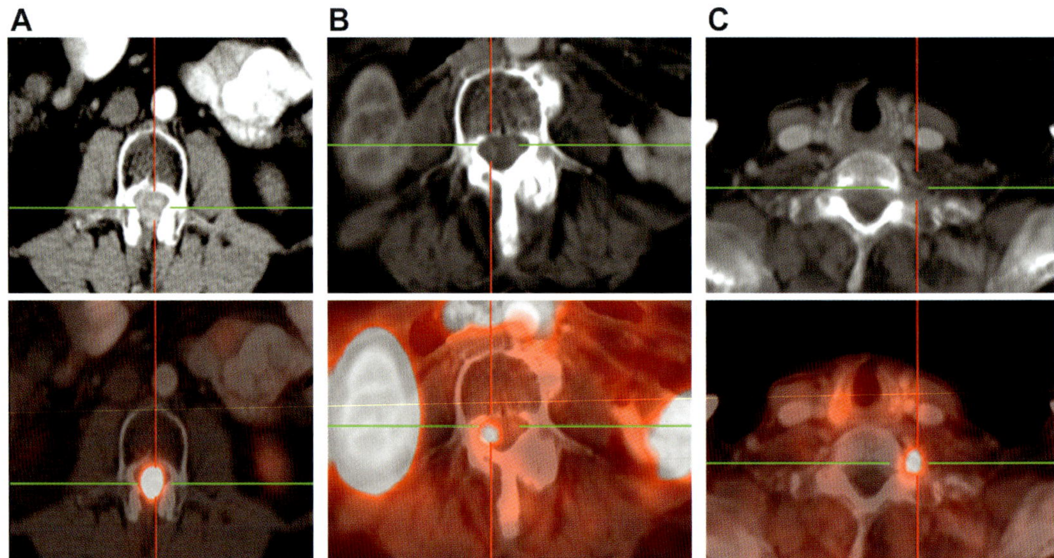

Fig. 3. Ga-68 DOTA-TATE PET/CT: Accuracy of disease localization. Intraspinal (*A, B*) and paravertebral (*C*) metastases of malignant pheochromocytoma.

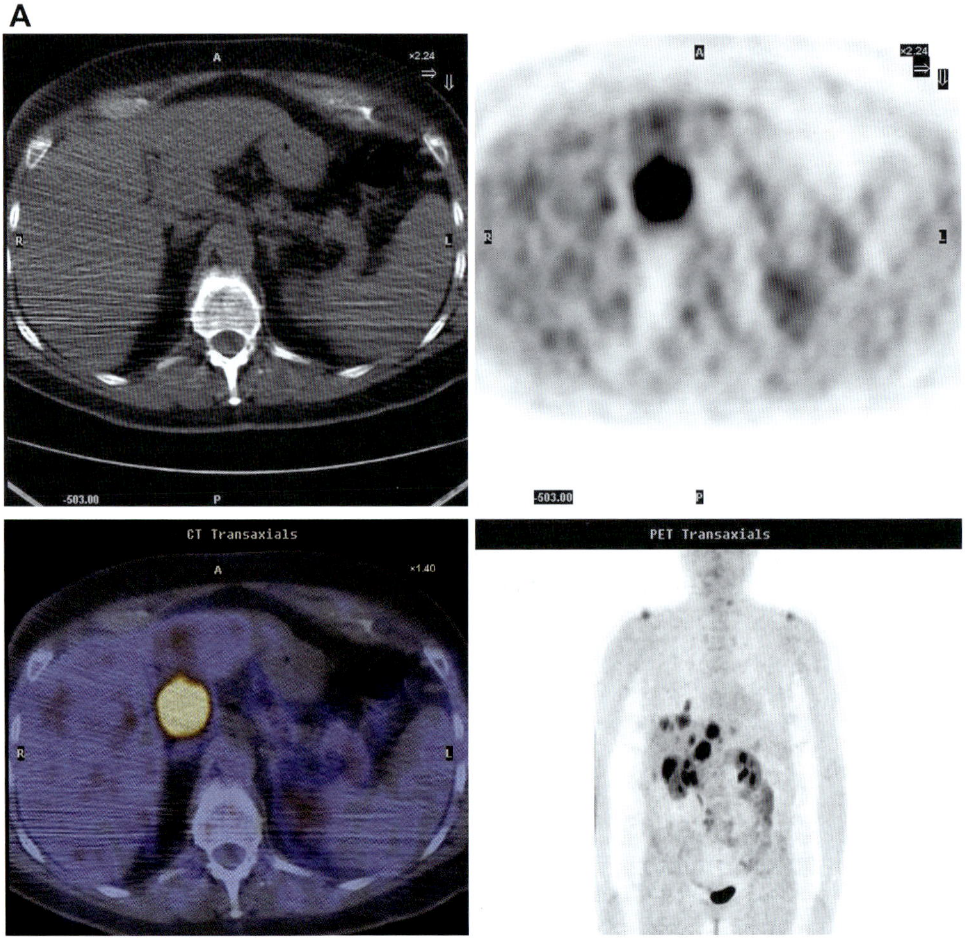

Fig. 4. ^{18}F-DOPA PET/CT images of a 63-year-old female with pancreatic NET. Indication to perform PET was initial staging. Conventional imaging showed peri-pancreatic nodes involvement, while SRS identified positive areas at liver level. ^{18}F-DOPA PET/CT images showed positive peri-pancreatic nodes (*A*), multiple liver metastasis (*B*) and sign of arthrosis.

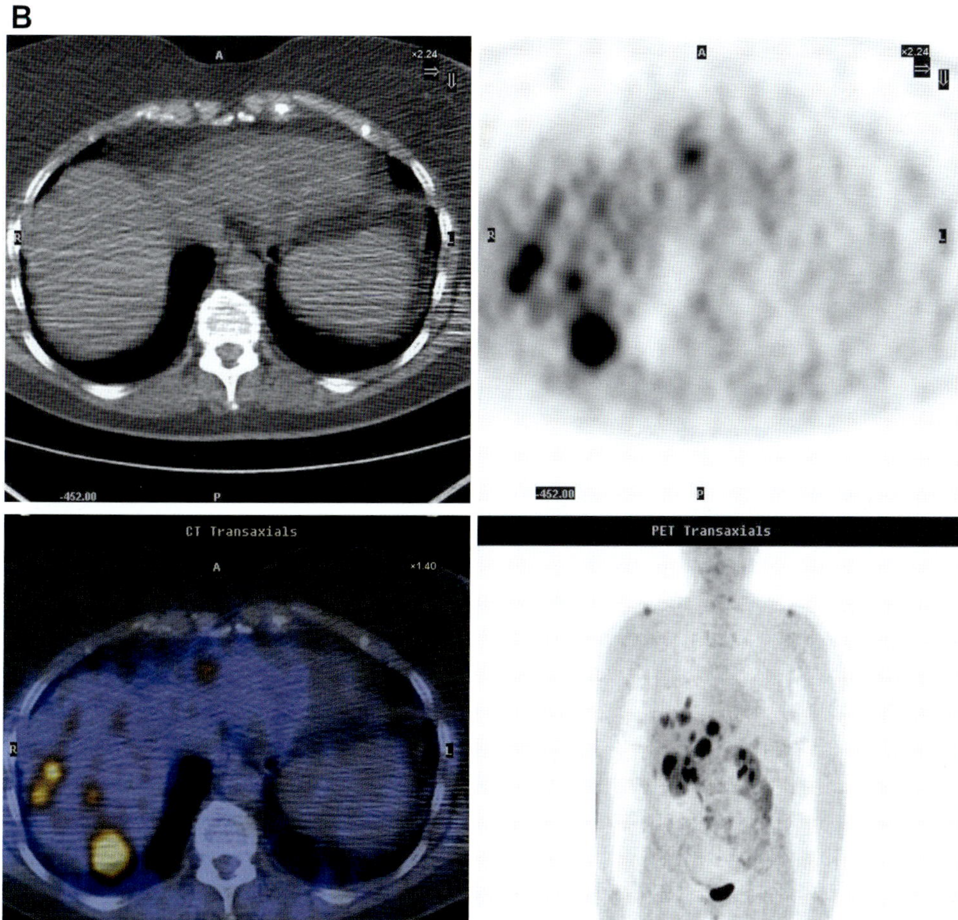

Fig. 4. (*continued*)

Metabolism-Targeted Radiopharmaceuticals

Pharmaceuticals that target the serotonin production pathway

Most of the clinical symptoms of a NET are caused by excessive production of serotonin. 5-Hydroxy-tryptophan is one of the intermediates in the production pathway that has been labeled successfully with [11]C.[29,30] A phase 1 clinical trial is underway to ascertain the role of ^{11}C-labeled-5-hydroxytryptophan in functional, serotonin-producing NETs.

Pharmaceuticals that target biogenic amine production and storage mechanism

NETs are characterized by the production and storage of several biogenic amines. One tracer with a design based on this observation is [11]C- or ^{18}F-labeled L-dihydroxyphenylalanine (DOPA). ^{18}F-DOPA is an aromatic amino acid labeled with [18]fluorine that was first used for the assessment of patients who have Parkinson's disease.[31] More recently, ^{18}F-DOPA has been used to differentiate between focal and diffuse congenital hyperglycemia[32] and study NETs. Belonging to the APUD (amine precursor uptake and decarboxylation) cells system, many NET cells avidly take up ^{18}F-DOPA and can be visualized by ^{18}F-DOPA-PET scans.

At the central and the peripheral nervous system level, ^{18}F-DOPA is transformed by COMT enzyme (Catechol-O-Methyl-Transferase) into Catechol-O-Methyl-fuloro-L-DOPA and by aromatic amino acid decarboxylase into 6-fluoro-dopamine (FDA).[33,34] Both products are then stored in secretory granules. Recent studies have demonstrated increased L-DOPA decarboxylase activity in 80% of NETs, and it has been suggested that this could be used as a marker of tumor activity.[35] Physiologic ^{18}F-DOPA uptake has been seen because of its excretion in the bile ducts, gallbladder, and digestive and urinary tracts.[36] Physiologic uptake in the striatum and pancreas has been reported.

Pharmaceuticals that target catecholamine transport pathway

Pheochromocytoma, neuroblastoma, and other chromaffin tissues concentrate many synthetic amine precursors using catecholamine transporters. ^{11}C-epinephrine (^{11}C-E) and ^{11}C hydroxy-epiphedrine (^{11}C-HED), both catecholamine analogs, and ^{18}F-fluorodopamine (^{18}F-FDA) are examples of such precursors (**Table 4**).[37]

Pharmaceuticals that target increased tumor glucose metabolism

One of the fundamental energy sources of many tumors is glucose. ^{18}F-2-fluoro-2-deoxyglucose (FDG) targets the glycolytic pathway, the main source of glucose consumption in tumors. FDG enters the glycolytic pathway like glucose in the cytoplasm, where it is phosphorylated by the enzyme hexokinase to FDG-6-phosphate. It does not get metabolized further, however, and gets trapped inside the neoplastic cells.

Imaging Protocols

Receptor positron emission tomography/CT using ^{68}Ga-DOTA-NOC

Sandostatin long-acting release injections must be stopped 4 to 6 weeks before the scan, and subcutaneous treatment with octreotide should be stopped at least 2 days before. Care should be taken to ensure that the patient is properly hydrated. Just before the acquisition, 1.5 L of an oral contrast dispersion, such as gastrografin, is given. PET/CT acquisition starts 60 minutes after intravenous injection of approximately 100 MBq (75–250 MBq) of the radiolabeled peptide ^{68}Ga-DOTA-NOC. To increase renal elimination and reduce radiation exposure to the urinary bladder, furosemide is given at the time of injection of ^{68}Ga-DOTA-NOC. Before the ^{68}Ga-DOTA-NOC PET acquisition, a low-dose, contrast-enhanced CT scan is performed. Protocol for CT scan is outlined in the SNM guidelines. Dynamic study gives more detailed and precise information about the kinetics of the radiopharmaceutical and allows absolute quantification.

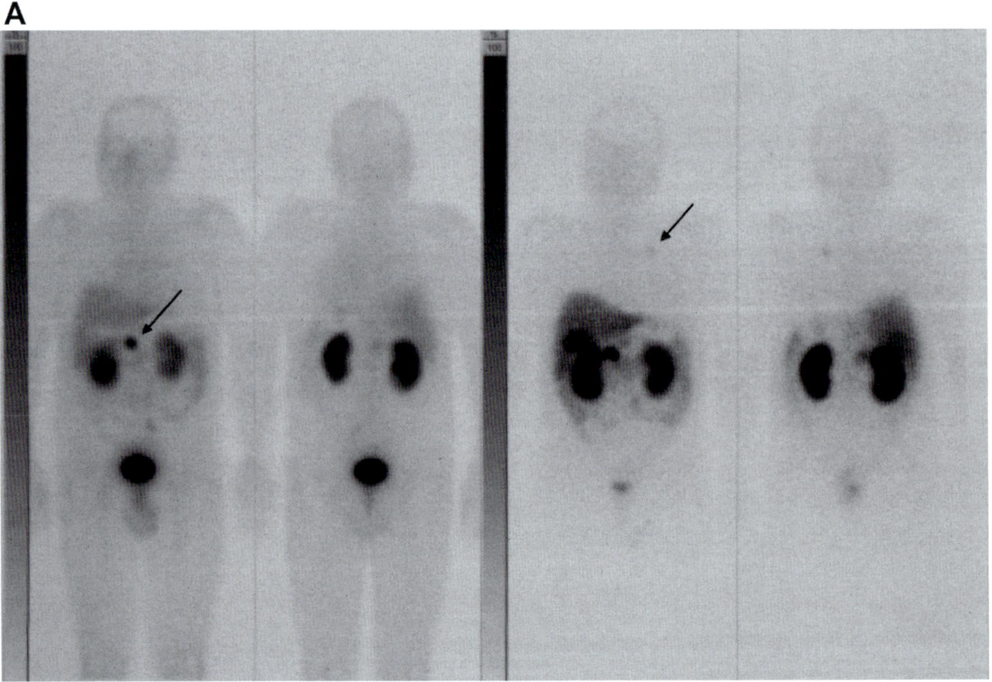

Fig. 5. ^{18}F-DOPA PET/CT images of a 60-year-old male with MEN1. Previous surgery: distal pancreatecomy. Conventional imaging showed a suspicious thoracic finding confirmed by SRS (A) that also detected the presence of intense uptake in the residual pancreas. (*Right arrow*) residual pancreas; (*Left arrow*) thoracic lesion. ^{18}F-DOPA PET/CT (B) confirmed the pathologic uptake at thoracic level (C) and also identified the presence of disease in the residual pancreas (D), although the reading of DOPA uptake at pancreas level is limited by the high physiologic uptake.

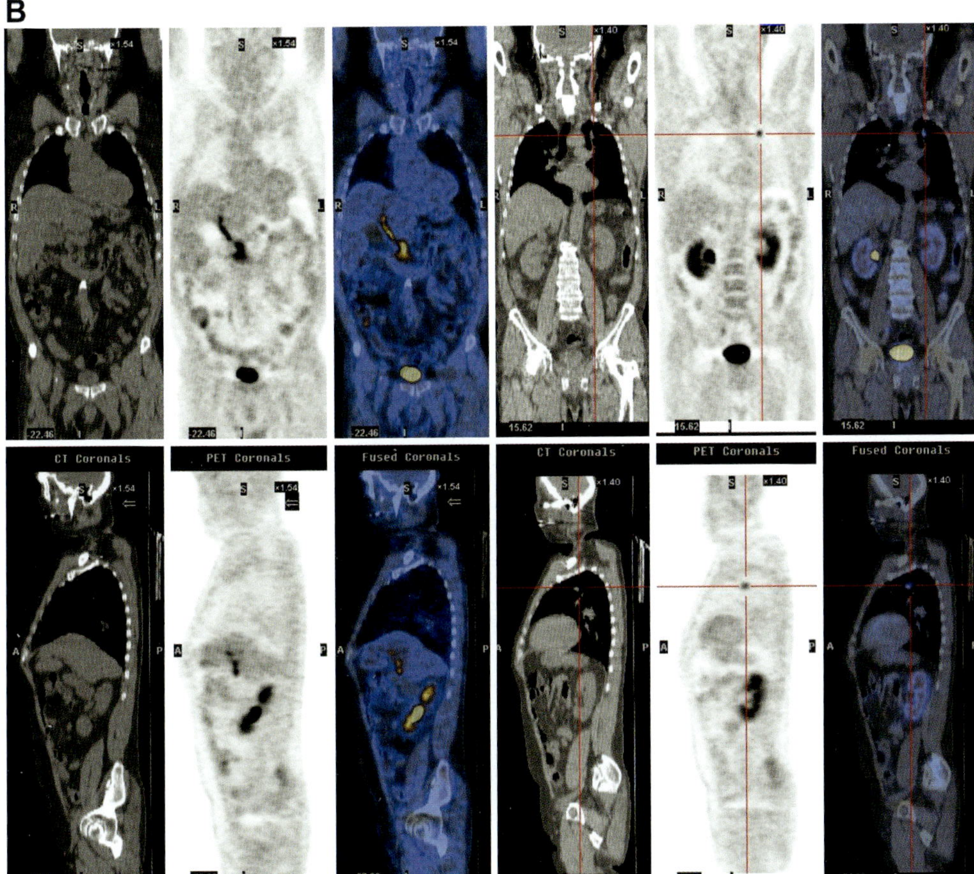

Fig. 5. (continued)

Biodistribution and dosimetry

The excretion of DOTA-NOC is primarily through the kidneys, which makes them the critical organs. The urinary bladder, spleen, and liver—in that order—also receive a high radiation dose. Overall, however ^{68}Ga-DOTA-NOC delivers a radiation dose to the organs comparable to, and even lower than, other diagnostic analogs. Despite the fact that DOTA-NOC covers the wider range of somatostatin receptors, this fact makes it an interesting and important approach. Other organs having known physiologic SSTR expression, such as the pituitary glands, and adrenals show mild to moderate uptake of DOTA-NOC.

Metabolic imaging protocol (F-18 DOPA-PET)

^{18}F-DOPA-PET is performed in patients who have fasted for 6 hours (intravenous injected dose: 5–6 MBq/kg, uptake time 60–90 min). It has been reported that the oral premedication with carbidopa, a peripheral aromatic amino acid decarboxylase inhibitor, enhances sensitivity by increasing the tumor-to-background ratio of tracer uptake.[38]

Carbidopa administration may be particularly useful for assessing lesions at sites with increased ^{18}F-DOPA physiologic uptake. Timmers and colleagues[39] recently described how premedication with carbidopa allowed visualization of three additional paraganglioma lesions that were undetected by ^{18}F-DOPA alone.

INDICATIONS FOR POSITRON EMISSION TOMOGRAPHY/CT
Diagnosis, Staging, and Restaging

Receptor positron emission tomography or positron emission tomography/CT

The variable nature, indolent course, and possibility of multiple and unpredictable primary anatomic sites make it difficult to evaluate patients with NETs. Until recently, ^{111}In-octreotide-SPECT has been considered to be the gold standard for NET diagnosis. Hofmann and colleagues[40] have shown that ^{68}Ga-DOTA-TOC is superior to ^{111}In-octreotide SPECT in detecting upper abdominal metastases when CT was taken as the reference for

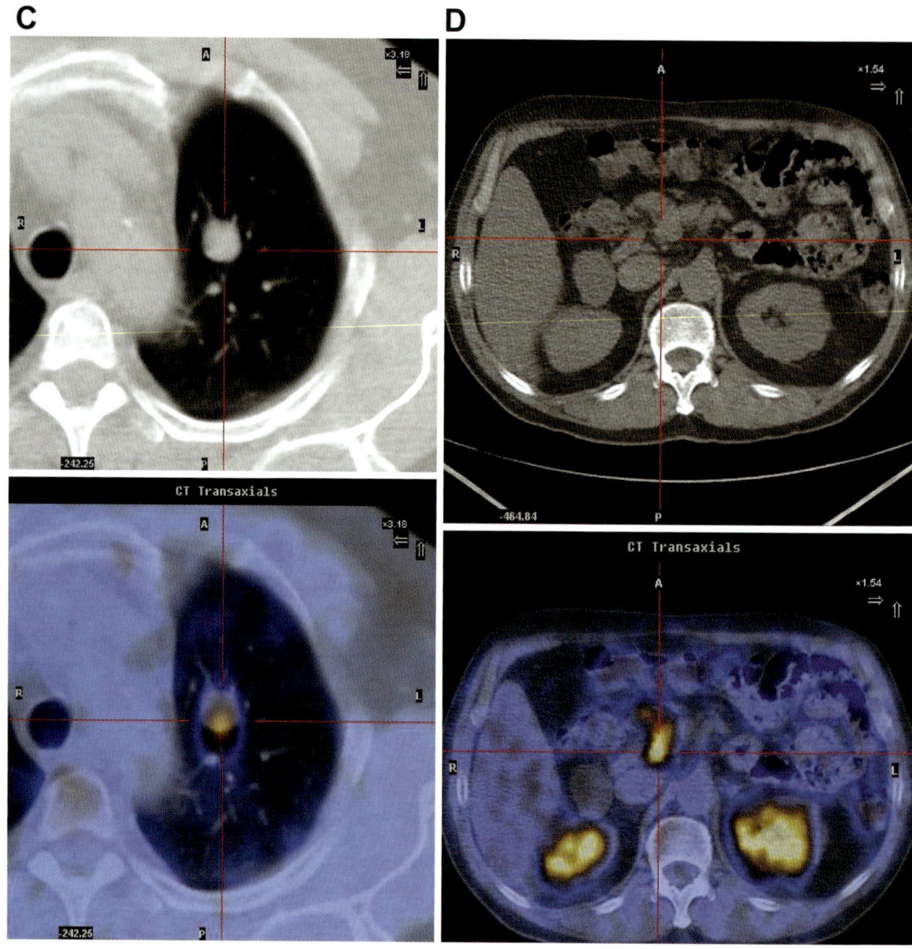

Fig. 5. (continued)

comparison. In a recent study by Buchmann and colleagues,[41] ^{68}Ga-DOTA-TOC PET/CT was proven to be superior to ^{111}In-DTPAOC in the detection of NET metastases to the lung and bone (Figs. 1–3).

In another study, Gabriel and colleagues[42] showed the feasibility and high accuracy of ^{68}Ga-DOTA-TOC PET as a promising tool for the detection of NET. The accuracy of PET (96%) was found to be significantly higher than that of CT (75%) and ^{111}In-DOTA-TOC SPECT (58%). In 32 patients, ^{68}Ga-DOTA-TOC PET was true positive, whereas SPECT results were false negative. PET also was able to detect more lesions than SPECT and CT. It was observed that for the staging of patients, PET was superior to CT or SPECT because it could pick up more lesions in lymph nodes, liver, and bone. Overall, PET provided additional clinically relevant information in 14% of patients when compared with SPECT and in 21% of patients when compared with CT. Other studies have validated these observations. Kowalski and colleagues[43] reported that ^{68}Ga-DOTA-TOC PET was superior to ^{111}In-octreotide imaging, especially in detecting small tumors or tumors bearing only a low density of somatostatin receptors. Apart from GEP tumors, ^{68}Ga-DOTA-TOC PET also has been envisioned to have a potential role in small-cell lung cancer because this tumor is known to express somatostatin receptors.[44]

In a study that compared the diagnostic efficacy of ^{68}Ga-DOTA-NOC and ^{68}Ga-DOTA-TATE in the same subject, Antunes and colleagues[45] demonstrated that ^{68}Ga-DOTA-NOC might be superior to ^{68}Ga-DOTA-TATE. Our experience with more than 2500 receptor PET/CT studies performed at the Zentralklinik Bad Berka shows clearly that ^{68}Ga-DOTA-NOC PET is able to detect many more lesions than CT. The independence of the somatostatin receptor state of the tumor from their metabolic activity (functionality) makes it possible to detect nonfunctional NET using receptor PET/CT.

PET using ^{68}Ga-DOTA-TOC has been found to be superior to F-18 FDG-PET in the detection of NET by detecting 90% of the lesions in 15 patients when compared with only 68% on FDG-PET.[46]

Gluc-Lys [(^{18}F)FP]-TOCA is another radiopharmaceutical that targets somatostatin receptors. In a preliminary comparative study, Gluc-Lys [(^{18}F)FP]-TOCA PET was found to be superior to ^{111}In-DTPA-octreotide scan in the diagnosis of NETs. The results also suggested that the sensitivity and specificity of Gluc-Lys [(^{18}F)FP]-TOCA are comparable to the reported sensitivity and specificity of ^{68}Ga-DOTA-TOC PET findings in NET.[47]

Another interesting radiopharmaceutical is ^{64}Cu-TETA-octreotide. [64]Cu (half-life 12.7 hours) has been shown to have great potential as a positron emitting radionuclide for PET imaging and radiotherapy.[48–51] The possibility of performing dosimetry for peptide receptor radionuclide therapy (PRRT) based on ^{64}Cu is one other possible advantage. In a preliminary study, ^{64}Cu-TETA-octreotide PET was found to have high sensitivity and favorable dosimetry and pharmacokinetics.[48]

Metabolic imaging

In recent years, studies have shown that ^{18}F-DOPA is useful for the assessment of NET and may be superior to conventional structural (US, CT, MR imaging) and somatostatin receptor scintigraphic (SRS) procedures, with sensitivities ranging from 65% to 100% (**Figs. 4–10**).[36,38,52–54]

In 2001, Hoegerle and colleagues[36] reported that ^{18}F-DOPA-PET detected a higher number of NET lesions in the gastrointestinal tract than SRS-based imaging or ^{18}F-FDG PET (true-positive findings at primary sites: 7 versus 4 versus 2; nodes metastasis: 41 versus 27 versus 14, respectively). In a prospective, single-center study, Koopmans and colleagues[38] compared ^{18}F-DOPA-PET results with SRS and CT in 53 patients with metastatic carcinoid tumor. ^{18}F-DOPA-PET was shown to have a higher sensitivity than SRS and CT alone (100% versus 92% and 87%, respectively) or when the latter two modalities were combined (96%). ^{18}F-DOPA-PET detected more lesions, more regions with lesions, and more lesions per region than SRS and CT.

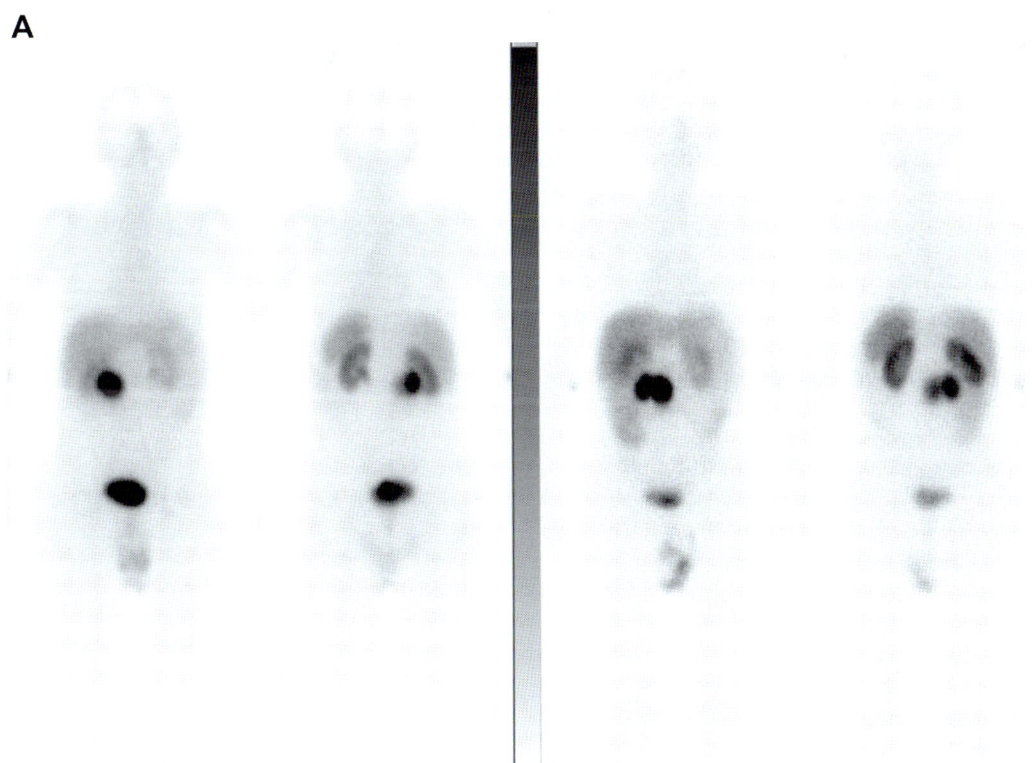

Fig. 6. ^{18}F-DOPA PET/CT images for staging of a 67-year old male with multiple duodenal gastrinomas with nodes metastasis (under therapy with sandostatin). Conventional imaging detected the presence of disease in the duodenum and at nodes level. SRS showed pathologic uptake only at nodes level (*A*) while PET/CT images identified the presence of both, pancreas (*B*) and positive nodes (*C*).

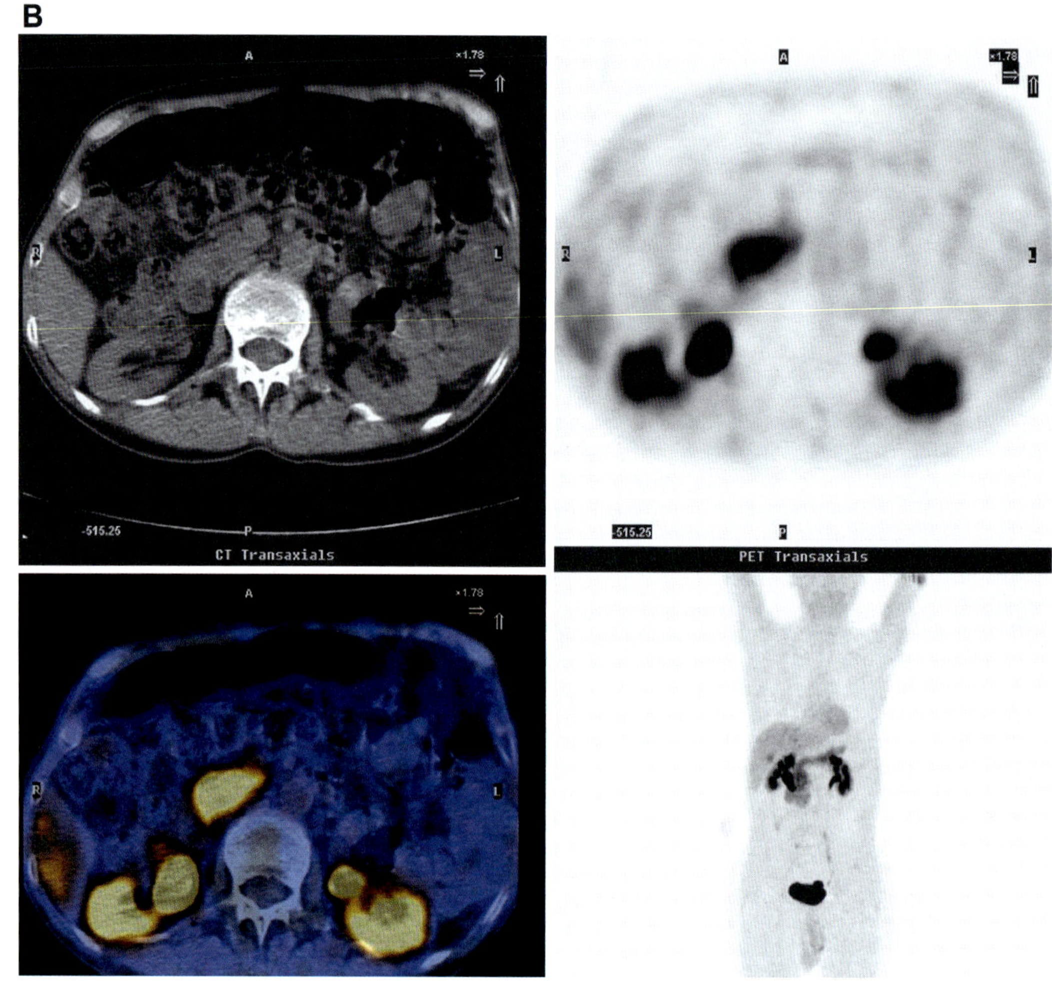

Fig. 6. (*continued*)

After imaging 23 advanced NET cases, Becherer and colleagues[52] reported that ^{18}F-DOPA-PET was more accurate than CT and SRS for the detection of NET, especially for bone lesions (^{18}F-DOPA sensitivity of 100% versus SRS sensitivity of 50%). The specificity of ^{18}F-DOPA-PET for the detection of liver involvement was 81% for skeletal disease 91%, and 100% for the abnormalities of the mediastinum, pancreas, and lymph nodes. Although wider availability, lower cost, and more specific mechanism of action render ^{68}Ga-DOTA peptides the tracers of choice for differentiated NET, ^{18}F-DOPA may offer advantages for the detection of tumors with a low or absent expression of SSR, such as medullary thyroid carcinoma[55] and undifferentiated NET. In 2001, Hoegerle and colleagues[56] reported good sensitivity for ^{18}F-DOPA-PET in medullar thyroid cancer (63%) with other imaging procedures (^{18}F-FDG-PET 44%, SRS 52%, morphologic imaging 82%).

The difficulty of interpreting the anatomic location of the primary tumor and the need to differentiate between scar tissue and local relapse of the primary tumor after surgery are major limitations of conventional imaging techniques in detecting thyroid carcinoma.

Currently, few studies have specifically investigated the role of ^{18}F-DOPA-PET in patients with medullary thyroid carcinoma, and the number of patients included in these studies is small. Findings on ^{18}F-DOPA scans were confirmed by either follow-up or pathology in only a few cases.[56–58]

Another condition in which ^{18}F-DOPA may offer advantages over ^{68}Ga-DOTA peptides is the assessment of adrenal neoplasms. Up to 50% of malignant pheochromocytomas and 15% of benign forms are undetected by CT, MR imaging, or ^{123}I-MIBG scans. Hoegerle and colleagues[53] and Mackenzie and colleagues[59] reported that

C

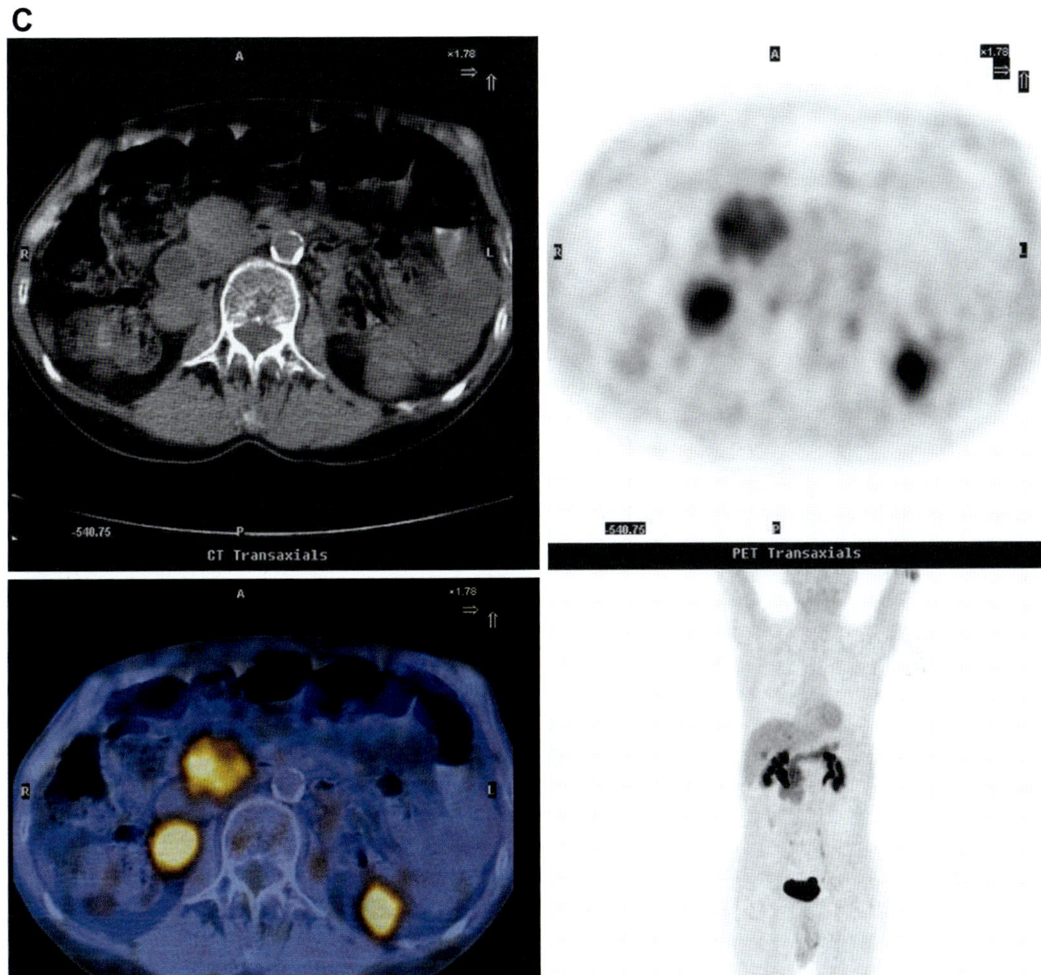

Fig. 6. *(continued)*

^{18}F-DOPA-PET can be particularly useful in these cases. ^{18}F-DOPA was also reported to be highly sensitive for the detection of glomus tumors.[60]

Regarding small-cell lung cancer, preliminary data in four patients suggested that ^{18}F-DOPA-PET is less accurate than FDG-PET and conventional imaging.[61] For this comparison, the agreement among FDG-PET, ^{18}F-DOPA-PET, and standard imaging procedures was made site by site. The results from ^{18}F-DOPA-PET and FDG-PET imaging were concordant in 4 out of 11 tumor sites, whereas FDG-PET and standard imaging procedures were in full agreement. ^{18}F-DOPA was negative in two of four cases in one study and in 7 of 11 sites in another study.

^{18}F-FDG positron emission tomography/CT

The use of FDG-PET in the diagnosis of NETs is limited to tumors that are undifferentiated and aggressive in nature.[29,62–66] It has been shown that FDG-PET is more sensitive than SSR (^{111}In-pentetreotide) in detecting poorly differentiated GEP tumors, but it was less sensitive in visualizing differentiated GEP tumors.[62] A multicenter study demonstrated that FDG-PET is a useful method for the staging and follow-up of patients with medullary thyroid cancer because it has the highest diagnostic accuracy compared with other imaging modalities, such as CT scan, SSR, and [99m]Tc(V) DMSA.[67]

[11]C-epinephrine, ^{11}C-hydroxyepiphedrine positron emission tomography

In neuroblastoma, Shulkin and colleagues[68] compared the role of ^{123}I-MIBG and ^{11}C-hydroxyepiphedrine (^{11}C-HED) PET and demonstrated that ^{11}C-HED-PET has high sensitivity for detecting neuroblastoma. Most of the tumor lesions visible on the ^{11}C-HED-PET also could be seen on ^{123}I-MIBG. One of the limitations of ^{11}C-HED-PET

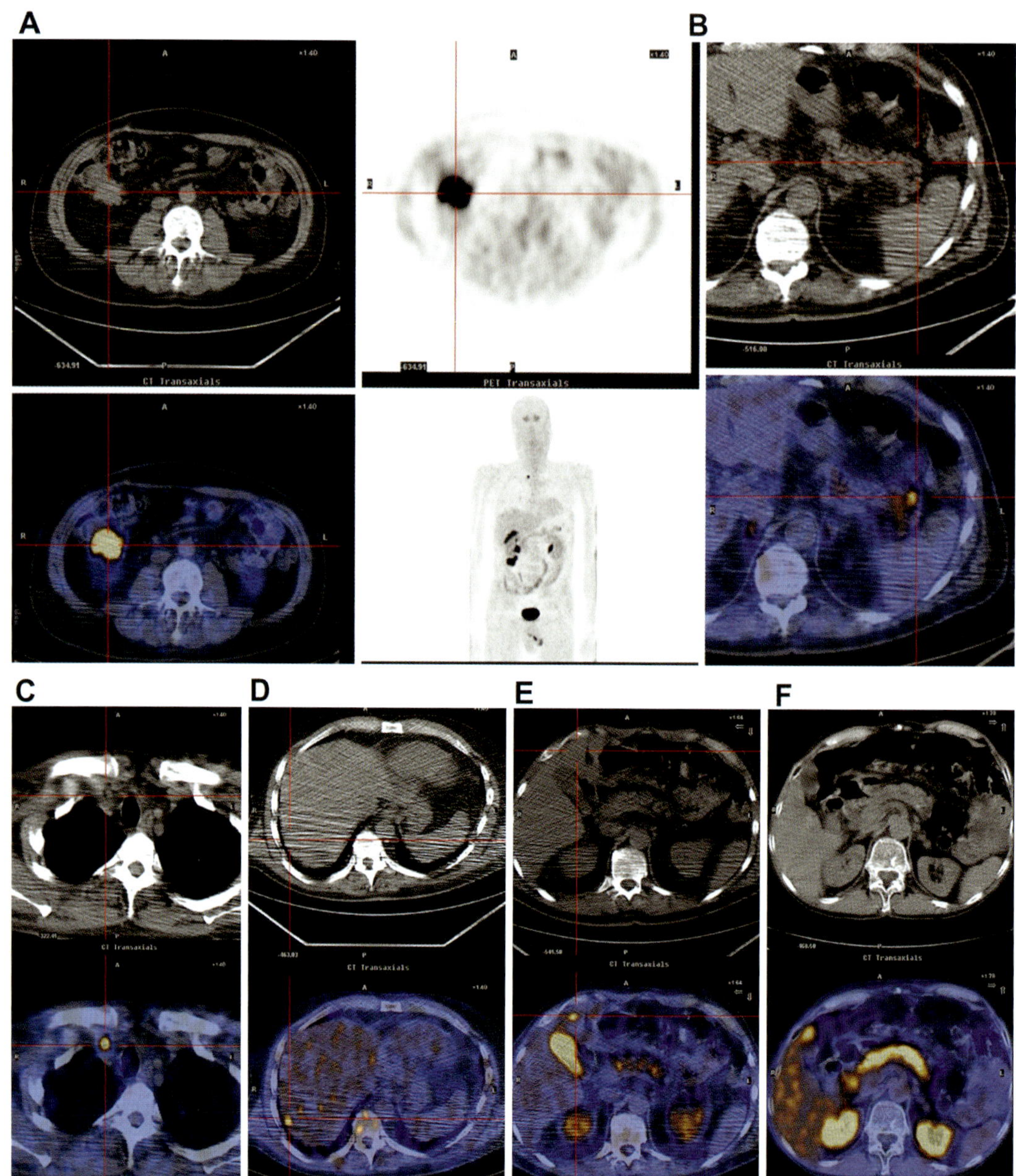

Fig. 7. ^{18}F-DOPA PET images of a 58-year old male with ileum NET investigated for re-staging. The normal physiologic distribution in the pancreas is often a hindrance in the detection of small pathologic lesion in the vicinity. Conventional imaging showed a solid mass at the ileo-cecal valve (*A*) while SRS was negative. PET/CT images confirmed the presence of a pathologic mass at the ileo-cecal valve level (SUV_{max} 14) and showed uptake in a small area in the pancreatic tail (*B*), in paratracheal nodes (SUV_{max} 9) (*C*) as well as multiple lesions in the liver (SUV_{max} 13) (*C, D*). 18F-DOPA physiologic pancreatic uptake is shown in (*E, F*).

was the high level of uptake in the liver, which is a source of error for localization of tumors in this organ. In another study conducted by the same group,[69] similar results were observed in ten patients with pheochromocytoma, which suggested a potential role of ^{11}C-HED. High cost, short half-life, and limited availability of ^{11}C have made wider clinical use of ^{11}C-HED impractical.

[11]C-epinephrine is also under evaluation and has the potential to be a potential agent for imaging neuroblastomas.

Detection of Unknown Primary Tumor

Receptor positron emission tomography/CT

Carcinoma of unknown primary origin is defined as a biopsy-proven secondary lesion with no

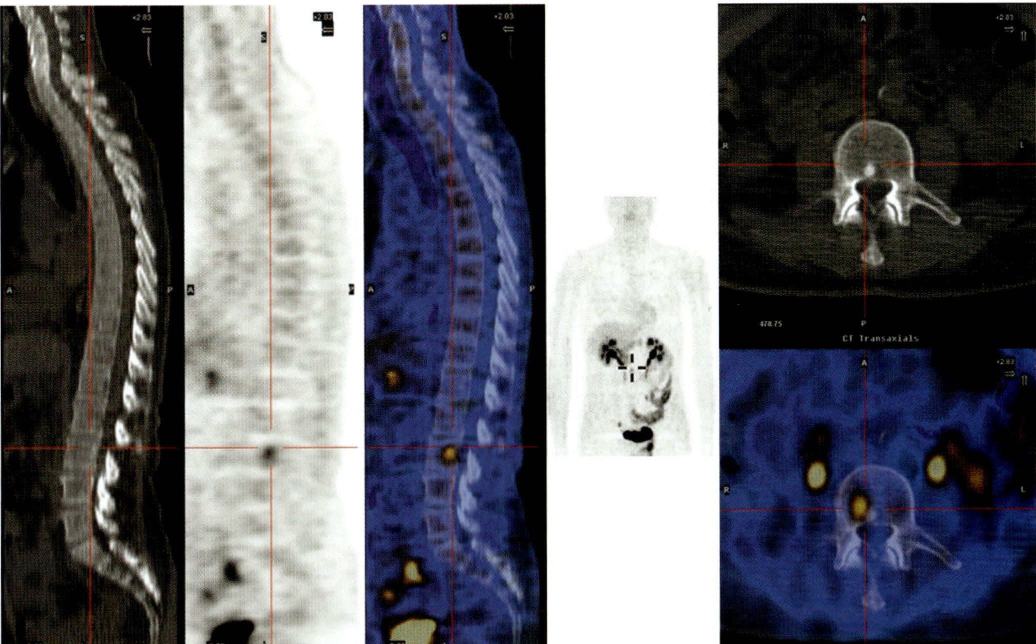

Fig. 8. ^{18}F-DOPA PET/CT images of a 72-year-old male with pancreatic NET (re-staging after surgery). Conventional imaging was inconclusive (US was negative while CT identified a suspicious lesion at L3 level) and SRS showed poorly defined somatostatin receptor positive lesions in the thoracic and abdomen. ^{18}F-DOPA PET/CT images confirmed the malignant nature of the L3 lesion and foci in the liver and pancreas.

detectable primary tumor after assessment by physical examination and conventional imaging tests (MR imaging, CT, and US). The site of the occult primary tumor may remain unidentified in a large number of patients after imaging with chest radiographs, abdominal and pelvic CT, and mammography in women or upon autopsy.[70–73] Overall, in approximately 3% of the patients, the site of origin of histologically documented carcinoma is not identified clinically. Lesion size smaller than the spatial resolution of the imaging modality being used, angiogenic incompetence leading to mass involution, and lesions in areas in which interpretation is difficult may account for the low detection rate.[74] The early identification of the primary tumor is

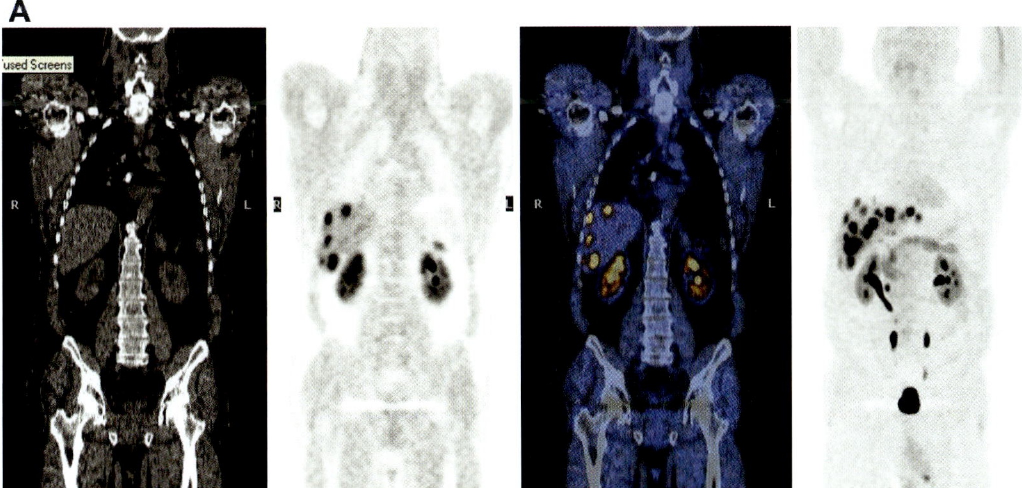

Fig. 9. ^{18}F-DOPA PET/CT images of a 75-year-old male with ileum NET (re-staging after surgery). Conventional imaging and SRS showed the presence of multiple liver metastases while ^{18}F-DOPA PET/CT confirmed the presence of liver metastasis (*A–C*) and also identified right mesenteric lymph node metastases (*D*).

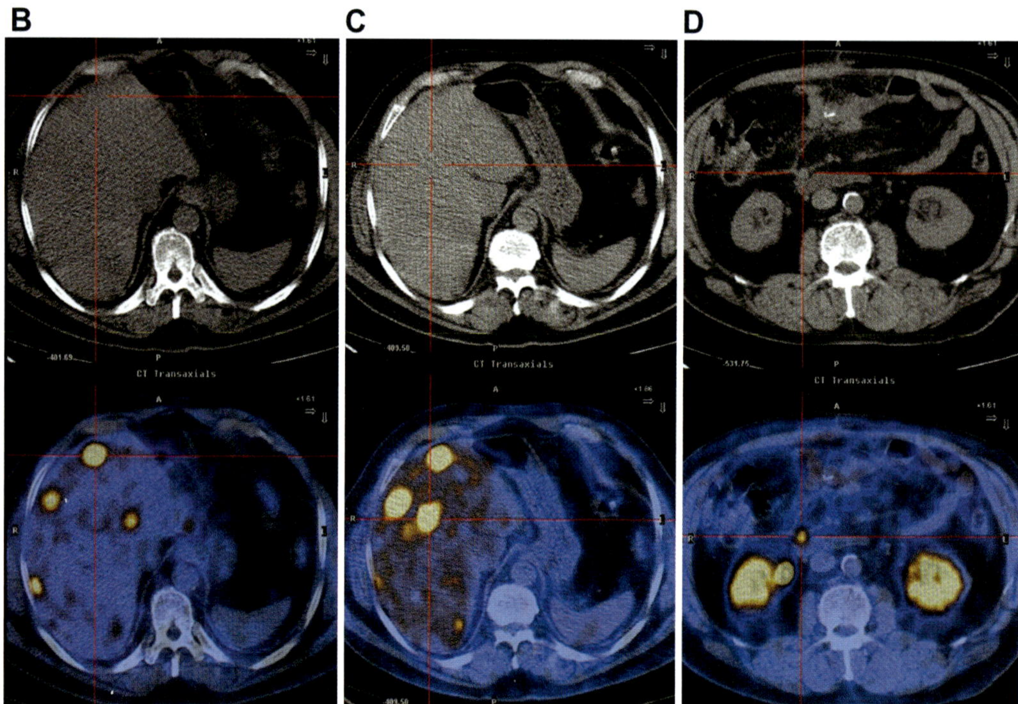

Fig. 9. (*continued*)

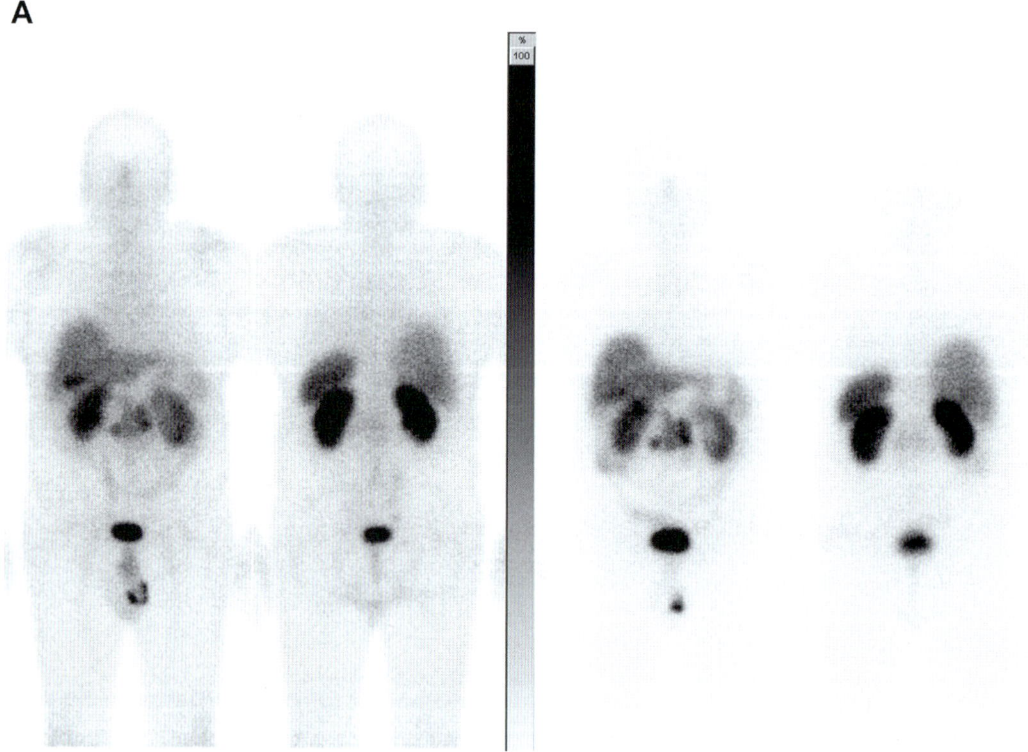

Fig. 10. ^{18}F-DOPA PET/CT images of a 64-year old male with ileum NET (re-staging after surgery) under sandostain therapy. Conventional imaging and SRS (*A*) showed the presence of abnormal peri-aortic nodes that were confirmed by ^{18}F-DOPA PET/CT (*B*) which, however, identified a larger number of lesions (multiple abdominal nodes and one supraclavicular node) (*C*).

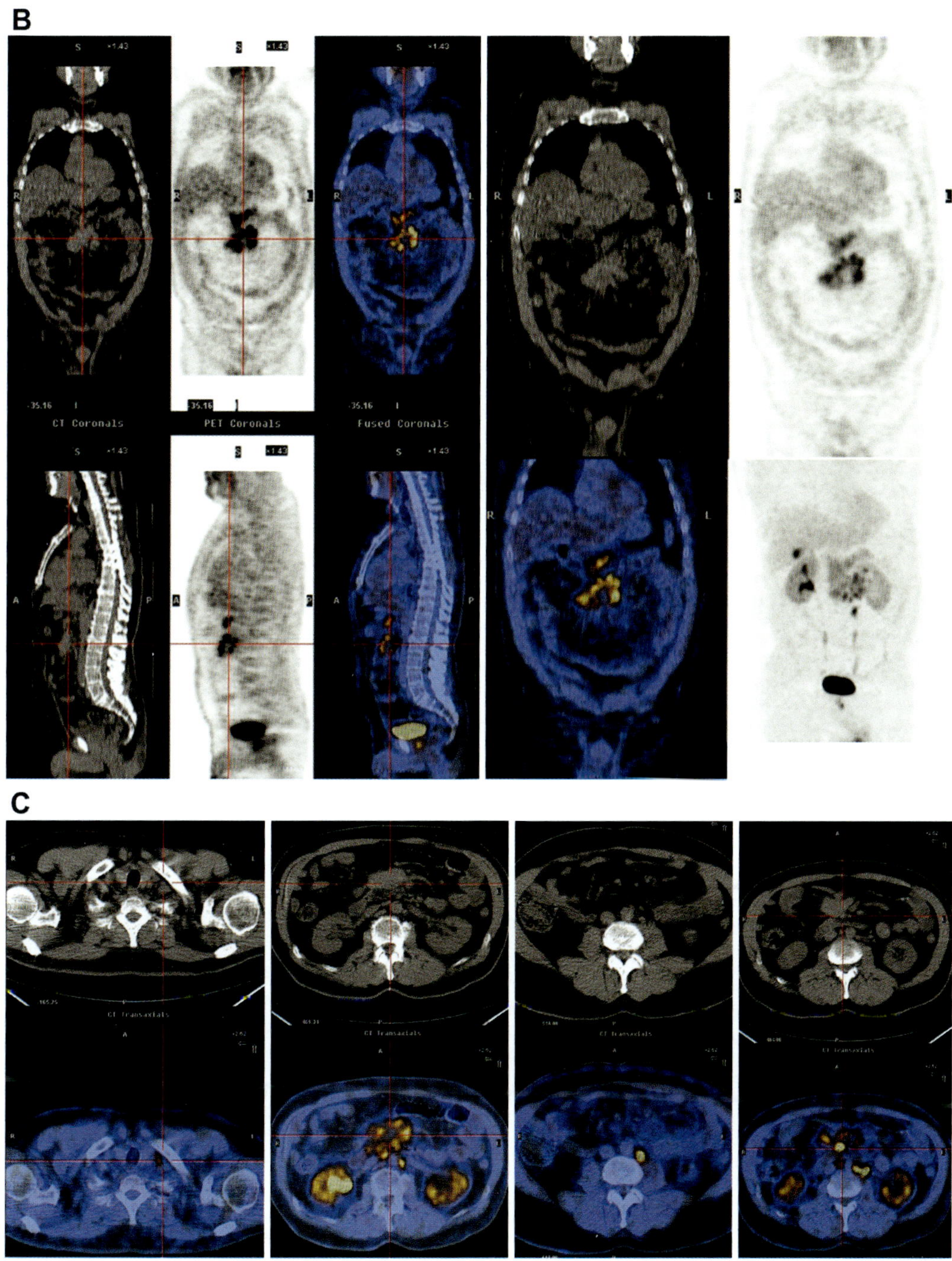

Fig. 10. (*continued*)

a fundamental requisite for predicting the prognosis and improving survival.[75] This is also true for NETs.

Whole-body PET/CT using FDG has been used successfully for the detection of the most common cancers that present as carcinoma of unknown primary origin, including adenocarcinomas, squamous cell carcinoma, and poorly differentiated carcinoma in which FDG-PET has identified the primary lesion in 24% to 40% of patients with negative conventional diagnostic investigations.[76–81] FDG-PET is of limited value in slow-growing, well-differentiated NETs, however.[62]

CT and MR imaging often fail to diagnose primary NET and endoscopic ultrasonography is limited to the detection of gastroenteropancreatic NET. These factors make receptor PET/CT imaging an indispensable tool in the initial diagnosis of the primary site and staging of patients with carcinoma of unknown primary origin.

Therapy Stratification

Curative treatment of NET usually requires complete surgical resection of the primary tumor and perhaps regional lymph nodes with proven metastases. Effective palliative therapies are also available at all stages of the disease, however, and are indicated even at advanced stages of their tumors. Depending on tumor stage, size, and degree of differentiation, current treatment protocols for NET include the following options:

1. Surgery
2. Immunologic therapy (interferon)
3. Intra-arterial chemoembolization
4. Chemotherapy
5. Therapy with somatostatin analogs
6. PRRT
7. ISIRT and RFTA

Surgical resection and cold somatostatin analogs (intramuscular or subcutaneous octreotide) are most commonly used as the first line of treatment; chemotherapy is used as the last option. Recent years have seen the development of PRRT as a highly effective treatment option for metastasized progressive NET, and this approach is regarded as the third option for this purpose. For effective management of patients who have NET, receptor and metabolic PET/CT play an important role.

By directing surgeons to the site of primary tumor, ^{68}Ga-DOTA-NOC and ^{18}F-DOPA-PET/CT improve the prognosis and quality of life for these patients. For cold somatostatin therapy and somatostatin receptor-based radionuclide therapy, it is essential to document the expression of these sites on the tumor cells. The therapy schedule (quantity of radiation and timing) of PRRT using ^{177}Lu or ^{90}Y-DOTA-TATE/DOTA-TOC depends highly on the semiquantitative or visual interpretation of ^{68}Ga-DOTA-NOC/DOTA-TOC-PET/CT. Although conventional dosimetry is important to individualize PRRT, in our own experience, semiquantitative (SUV_{max}) evaluation seems to predict the degree of receptor concentration and response (**Figs. 11, 12**).

Intra-arterial PRRT is an option, partial hepatectomy, and SIRT are other possible options. The dose to be administered for such treatments also depends on receptor expression because size on CT and MR imaging is not a reliable parameter because of the possibility of cystic degeneration and other nonfunctional tissues in the tumor.

Ambrosini and colleagues[82] also reported that in a limited population of biopsy-proven NET, ^{18}F-DOPA-PET offered relevant information for the clinical management of patients with an unclear clinical presentation or with inconclusive findings on other imaging modalities (US, CT, SRS, MR imaging). In particular, ^{18}F-DOPA-PET changed patient management in 11 of 13 cases.

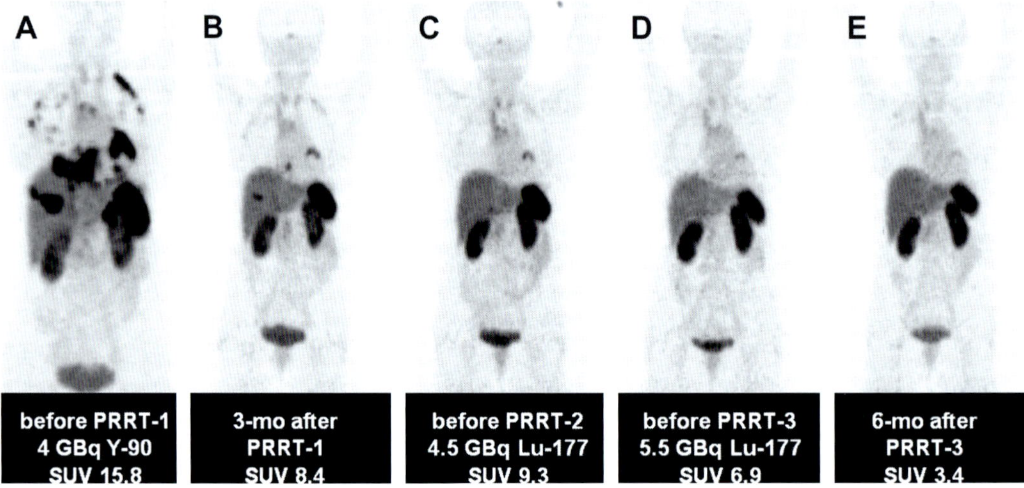

Fig. 11. Ga-68 DOTA-NOC PET/CT: MIP images (*A–E*) for evaluating therapy response by visual assessment in a patient with metastatic mediastinal NET (most probably arising from the thymus) under sequential PRRT using Y-90 and Lu-177 DOTA-TATE.

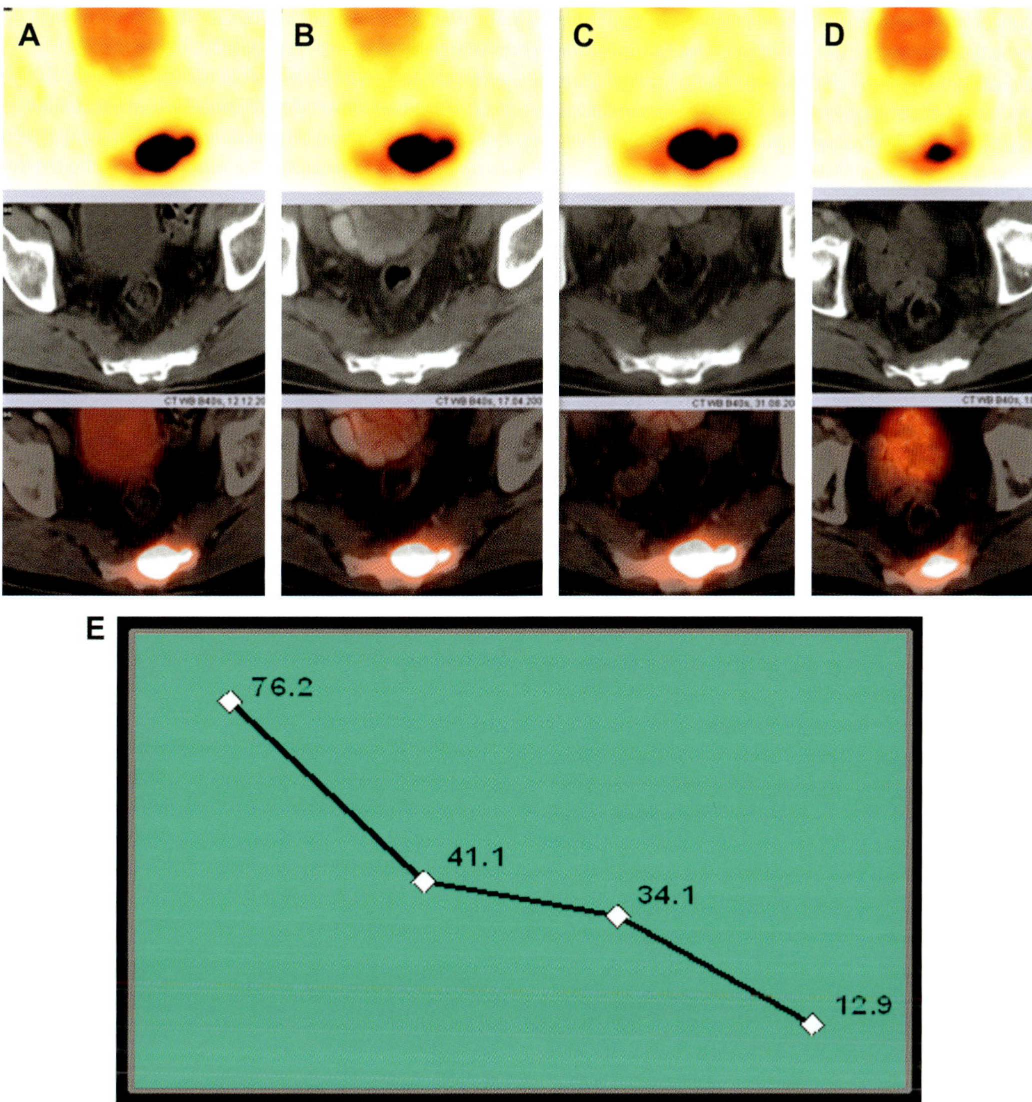

Fig. 12. Ga-68 DOTA-TATE PET/CT: Presacral paraganglioma with sacral invasion presenting with bone, liver and lymph node metastases, progressive at baseline (*A*) and responding well to peptide receptor radionuclide therapy (PRRT) administering three courses (*B–D*) of Y-90 and Lu-177 DOTA-TATE (total activity applied: 13,3 GBq). Time course of SUVmax of the presacral paraganglioma is also shown (*E*), dropping from 76.2 to 12.9 (partial response). Clinically dramatic pain reduction (the patient needed high doses of morphine before treatment and could give up completely on pain medication). Please mind that there is only little change on concurrent CT scan ("molecular response preceeds anatomical changes").

Further surgery, other than that necessary to remove the primary tumor, was avoided in four cases. In three patients, a surgical extirpation of the metabolic lesion was guided by ^{18}F-DOPA-PET/CT findings, and in four nonoperable patients with bone marrow metastasis, chemotherapy was administered. One patient with a false-positive PET result had a lymph node removed and remained disease free during follow-up.

FDG-PET was noted to have the potential to change the treatment protocol in 17% of patients who had pancreatic-duodenal NETs. FDG-PET was best suited for patients suspected of having a malignant tumor or a pancreatic mass larger than 2 cm or a case of multiple neuroendocrine neoplasia I with at least one visible lesion. The authors also reported that FDG-PET is not useful in duodenal tumors, benign insulinomas, and small, single pancreatic neuroendocrine lesions.[83]

Evaluation of Therapy Response

PET/CT is increasingly being used for monitoring response to therapy for various tumors. Until recently, the response parameters have been based on morphologic images. Recently, however, the use of molecular response criteria for the early and accurate detection of response to therapy has gained great interest in medical and surgical oncology.

ROLE OF METABOLIC POSITRON EMISSION TOMOGRAPHY/CT

The role of metabolic PET/CT imaging techniques in the assessment of response to therapy is almost nonexistent, primarily because NETs are slow-growing tumors and no definitive therapy exists that influences cellular metabolism directly enough to be assessed by FDG or ^{18}F-DOPA-PET/CT. In a preliminary study at the Zentralklinik Bad Berka, ^{68}Ga-DOTA-NOC-PET/CT was found to be superior to FDG-PET/CT for the early and accurate prediction of response to PRRT.[84] More data are needed to substantiate this observation, however. The other potential application of receptor and metabolic PET/CT would be in the assessment of response to transarterial chemoembolization, chemotherapy, and sandostatin therapy (to predict relapse). Biochemical markers are not good indicators for early and accurate response to therapy, which further emphasizes the need to establish the role of PET/CT in the monitoring of treatment response.

REFERENCES

1. Oberndorfer S. Karzinoidtumore des Dünndarms. Frankf Z Pathol 1907;1:426–9.
2. Vinik AI, Woltering EA, O'Dorisio TM, et al. Neuroendocrine tumors: a comprehensive guide to diagnosis and management. Inter Science Institute; 2006.
3. Jensen RT. Endocrine tumors of the gastrointestinal tract and pancreas. In: Kasper DL, Fauci AS, Longo DL, et al, editors. Harrison's principles of internal medicine. 16th edition. McGraw-Hill; 2005. p. 2347–58.
4. Schmitt-Gräff A, Hezel B, Wiedenmann B. Pathologisch-diagnostische Aspekte neuroendokriner Tumoren des Gastrointestinaltrakts. Der Onkologe 2000;613–23.
5. Solcia E, Kloppel G, Sobin LH. Histological typing of tumors: international histological classification of tumors in collaboration with 9 pathologists from 4 countries. In: Organisation WHOPPWH. 2nd edition.. Berlin (Germany): Springer; 2000.
6. Rindi G, Kloppel G, Alhman H, et al. TNM staging of foregut (neuro)endocrine tumors: a consensus proposal including a grading system. Virchows Arch 2006;449:395–401.
7. Reubi JC. Peptide receptors as molecular targets for cancer diagnosis and therapy. Endocr Rev 2003;24: 389–427.
8. Reubi JC, Schar JC, Waser B, et al. Affinity profiles for human somatostatin receptor subtypes SST1-SST5 of somatostatin radiotracers selected for scintigraphic and radiotherapeutic use. Eur J Nucl Med 2000;27:273–82.
9. Reubi JC, Waser B, Schaer JC, et al. Somatostatin receptor sst1-sst5 expression in normal and neoplastic human tissues using receptor autoradiography with subtype-selective ligands. Eur J Nucl Med 2001;28:836–46.
10. Rufini V, Calcagni ML, Baum RP. Imaging of neuroendocrine tumors. Semin Nucl Med 2006;36: 228–47.
11. Wild D, Macke HR, Waser B, et al. 68Ga-DOTANOC: a first compound for PET imaging with high affinity for somatostatin receptor subtypes 2 and 5. Eur J Nucl Med Mol Imaging 2005;32:724.
12. Wild D, Schmitt JS, Ginj M, et al. DOTA-NOC, a high-affinity ligand of somatostatin receptor subtypes 2, 3 and 5 for labelling with various radiometals. Eur J Nucl Med Mol Imaging 2003;30:1338–47.
13. Ginj M, Zhang H, Waser B, et al. Radiolabeled somatostatin receptor antagonists are preferable to agonists for in vivo peptide receptor targeting of tumors. Proc Natl Acad Sci USA 2006;103:16436–41.
14. Reubi JC, Schaer JC, Wenger S, et al. SST3-selective potent peptidic somatostatin receptor antagonists. Proc Natl Acad Sci USA 2000;97:13973–8.
15. Rösch F, Knapp WH. In: Radionuclide generators, vol. 4. Rotterdam (The Netherlands): Kluwer Academic Publishers; 2003.
16. Zhernosekov KP, Filosofov DV, Baum RP, et al. Processing of generator-produced 68Ga for medical application. J Nucl Med 2007;48:1741–8.
17. Meyer GJ, Macke H, Schuhmacher J, et al. 68Ga-labelled DOTA-derivatised peptide ligands. Eur J Nucl Med Mol Imaging 2004;31:1097–104.
18. Moody TW, Hill JM, Jensen RT. VIP as a trophic factor in the CNS and cancer cells. Peptides 2003; 24:163–77.
19. Reubi JC, Waser B. Concomitant expression of several peptide receptors in neuroendocrine tumours: molecular basis for in vivo multireceptor tumour targeting. Eur J Nucl Med Mol Imaging 2003;30:781–93.
20. Thakur ML, Marcus CS, Saeed S, et al. 99mTc-labeled vasoactive intestinal peptide analog for rapid localization of tumors in humans. J Nucl Med 2000;41:107–10.
21. Virgolini I, Kurtaran A, Raderer M, et al. Vasoactive intestinal peptide receptor scintigraphy. J Nucl Med 1995;36:1732–9.
22. Virgolini I, Raderer M, Kurtaran A, et al. Vasoactive intestinal peptide-receptor imaging for the

localization of intestinal adenocarcinomas and endocrine tumors. N Engl J Med 1994;331:1116–21.

23. Behe M, Becker W, Gotthardt M, et al. Improved kinetic stability of DTPA- dGlu as compared with conventional monofunctional DTPA in chelating indium and yttrium: preclinical and initial clinical evaluation of radiometal labelled minigastrin derivatives. Eur J Nucl Med Mol Imaging 2003;30:1140–6.

24. Behr TM, Behe M, Angerstein C, et al. Cholecystokinin-B/gastrin receptor binding peptides: preclinical development and evaluation of their diagnostic and therapeutic potential. Clin Cancer Res 1999;5: 3124s–38s.

25. Behr TM, Jenner N, Radetzky S, et al. Targeting of cholecystokinin-B/gastrin receptors in vivo: preclinical and initial clinical evaluation of the diagnostic and therapeutic potential of radiolabelled gastrin. Eur J Nucl Med 1998;25:424–30.

26. Breeman WA, De Jong M, Bernard BF, et al. Pre-clinical evaluation of [(111)In-DTPA-Pro(1), Tyr(4)]bombesin, a new radioligand for bombesin-receptor scintigraphy. Int J Cancer 1999;83:657–63.

27. Kwekkeboom DJ, Bakker WH, Kooij PP, et al. Cholecystokinin receptor imaging using an octapeptide DTPA-CCK analogue in patients with medullary thyroid carcinoma. Eur J Nucl Med 2000;27:1312–7.

28. Reubi JC, Waser B, Schaer JC, et al. Unsulfated DTPA- and DOTA-CCK analogs as specific high-affinity ligands for CCK-B receptor-expressing human and rat tissues in vitro and in vivo. Eur J Nucl Med 1998;25:481–90.

29. Eriksson B, Bergstrom M, Orlefors H, et al. Use of PET in neuroendocrine tumors: in vivo applications and in vitro studies. Q J Nucl Med 2000;44:68–76.

30. Orlefors H, Sundin A, Ahlstrom H, et al. Positron emission tomography with 5-hydroxytryprophan in neuroendocrine tumors. J Clin Oncol 1998;16:2534–41.

31. Eidelberg D, Moeller JR, Dhawan V, et al. The metabolic anatomy of Parkinson's disease: complementary [18F]fluorodeoxyglucose and [18F]fluorodopa positron emission tomographic studies. Mov Disord 1990;5:203–13.

32. Ribeiro MJ, Boddaert N, Bellanne-Chantelot C, et al. The added value of [(18)F]fluoro-L-DOPA PET in the diagnosis of hyperinsulinism of infancy: a retrospective study involving 49 children. Eur J Nucl Med Mol Imaging 2007;34:2120–8.

33. Creveling CR, Kirk KL. The effect of ring-fluorination on the rate of O-methylation of dihydroxyphenylalanine (DOPA) by catechol-O-methyltransferase: significance in the development of 18F-PET scanning agents. Biochem Biophys Res Commun 1985;130: 1123–31.

34. Melega WP, Luxen A, Perlmutter MM, et al. Comparative in vivo metabolism of 6-[18F]fluoro-L-dopa and [3H]L-dopa in rats. Biochem Pharmacol 1990;39: 1853–60.

35. Eldrup E, Clausen N, Scherling B, et al. Evaluation of plasma 3,4-dihydroxyphenylacetic acid (DOPAC) and plasma 3,4-dihydroxyphenylalanine (DOPA) as tumor markers in children with neuroblastoma. Scand J Clin Lab Invest 2001;61: 479–90.

36. Hoegerle S, Altehoefer C, Ghanem N, et al. Whole-body 18F DOPA PET for detection of gastrointestinal carcinoid tumors. Radiology 2001;220:373–80.

37. Kolby L, Bernhardt P, Levin-Jakobsen AM, et al. Uptake of meta-iodobenzylguanidine in neuroendocrine tumours is mediated by vesicular monoamine transporters. Br J Cancer 2003;89:1383–8.

38. Koopmans KP, de Vries EG, Kema IP, et al. Staging of carcinoid tumours with 18F-DOPA PET: a prospective, diagnostic accuracy study. Lancet Oncol 2006; 7:728–34.

39. Timmers HJ, Hadi M, Carrasquillo JA, et al. The effects of carbidopa on uptake of 6-18F-fluoro-L-DOPA in PET of pheochromocytoma and extraadrenal abdominal paraganglioma. J Nucl Med 2007;48:1599–606.

40. Hofmann M, Maecke H, Borner R, et al. Biokinetics and imaging with the somatostatin receptor PET radioligand (68)Ga-DOTATOC: preliminary data. Eur J Nucl Med 2001;28:1751–7.

41. Buchmann I, Henze M, Engelbrecht S, et al. Comparison of 68Ga-DOTATOC PET and 111In-DTPAOC (Octreoscan) SPECT in patients with neuroendocrine tumours. Eur J Nucl Med Mol Imaging 2007; 34:1617–26.

42. Gabriel M, Decristoforo C, Kendler D, et al. 68Ga-DOTA-Tyr3-octreotide PET in neuroendocrine tumors: comparison with somatostatin receptor scintigraphy and CT. J Nucl Med 2007; 48:508–18.

43. Kowalski J, Henze M, Schuhmacher J, et al. Evaluation of positron emission tomography imaging using [68Ga]-DOTA-D Phe(1)-Tyr(3)-Octreotide in comparison to [111In]-DTPAOC SPECT: first results in patients with neuroendocrine tumors. Mol Imaging Biol 2003;5:42–8.

44. Maecke HR, Hofmann M, Haberkorn U. (68)Ga-labeled peptides in tumor imaging. J Nucl Med 2005;46(Suppl 1):172S–8S.

45. Antunes P, Ginj M, Zhang H, et al. Are radiogallium-labelled DOTA-conjugated somatostatin analogues superior to those labelled with other radiometals? Eur J Nucl Med Mol Imaging 2007;982–93.

46. Koukouraki S, Strauss LG, Georgoulias V, et al. Evaluation of the pharmacokinetics of 68Ga-DOTATOC in patients with metastatic neuroendocrine tumours scheduled for 90Y-DOTATOC therapy. Eur J Nucl Med Mol Imaging 2006;33:460–6.

47. Meisetschlager G, Poethko T, Stahl A, et al. Gluc-Lys([18F]FP)-TOCA PET in patients with SSTR-positive tumors: biodistribution and diagnostic

evaluation compared with [111In]DTPA-octreotide. J Nucl Med 2006;47:566–73.

48. Anderson CJ, Dehdashti F, Cutler PD, et al. 64Cu-TETA-octreotide as a PET imaging agent for patients with neuroendocrine tumors. J Nucl Med 2001;42:213–21.

49. Lewis JS, Lewis MR, Cutler PD, et al. Radiotherapy and dosimetry of 64Cu-TETA-Tyr3-octreotate in a somatostatin receptor-positive, tumor-bearing rat model. Clin Cancer Res 1999;5:3608–16.

50. Sprague JE, Peng Y, Sun X, et al. Preparation and biological evaluation of copper-64-labeled tyr3-octreotate using a cross-bridged macrocyclic chelator. Clin Cancer Res 2004;10:8674–82.

51. Wang M, Caruano AL, Lewis MR, et al. Subcellular localization of radiolabeled somatostatin analogues: implications for targeted radiotherapy of cancer. Cancer Res 2003;63:6864–9.

52. Becherer A, Szabo M, Karanikas G, et al. Imaging of advanced neuroendocrine tumors with (18)F-FDOPA PET. J Nucl Med 2004;45:1161–7.

53. Hoegerle S, Nitzsche E, Altehoefer C, et al. Pheochromocytomas: detection with 18F DOPA whole body PET: initial results. Radiology 2002;222:507–12.

54. Nanni C, Fanti S, Rubello D. 18F-DOPA PET and PET/CT. J Nucl Med 2007;48:1577–9.

55. Reubi JC, Chayvialle JA, Franc B, et al. Somatostatin receptors and somatostatin content in medullary thyroid carcinomas. Lab Invest 1991;64:567–73.

56. Hoegerle S, Altehoefer C, Ghanem N, et al. 18F-DOPA positron emission tomography for tumour detection in patients with medullary thyroid carcinoma and elevated calcitonin levels. Eur J Nucl Med 2001;28:64–71.

57. Beuthien-Baumann B, Strumpf A, Zessin J, et al. Diagnostic impact of PET with 18F-FDG, 18F-DOPA and 3-O-methyl-6-[18F]fluoro-DOPA in recurrent or metastatic medullary thyroid carcinoma. Eur J Nucl Med Mol Imaging 2007;34:1604–9.

58. Crippa F, Alessi A, Gerali A, et al. FDG-PET in thyroid cancer. Tumori 2003;89:540–3.

59. Mackenzie IS, Gurnell M, Balan KK, et al. The use of 18-fluoro-dihydroxyphenylalanine and 18-fluorodeoxyglucose positron emission tomography scanning in the assessment of metaiodobenzylguanidine-negative phaeochromocytoma. Eur J Endocrinol 2007;157:533–7.

60. Hoegerle S, Ghanem N, Altehoefer C, et al. 18F-DOPA positron emission tomography for the detection of glomus tumours. Eur J Nucl Med Mol Imaging 2003;30:689–94.

61. Jacob T, Grahek D, Younsi N, et al. Positron emission tomography with [(18)F]FDOPA and [(18)F]FDG in the imaging of small cell lung carcinoma: preliminary results. Eur J Nucl Med Mol Imaging 2003;30:1266–9.

62. Adams S, Baum R, Rink T, et al. Limited value of fluorine-18 fluorodeoxyglucose positron emission tomography for the imaging of neuroendocrine tumours. Eur J Nucl Med 1998;25:79–83.

63. Pasquali C, Rubello D, Sperti C, et al. Neuroendocrine tumor imaging: can 18F-fluorodeoxyglucose positron emission tomography detect tumors with poor prognosis and aggressive behavior? World J Surg 1998;22:588–92.

64. Scanga DR, Martin WH, Delbeke D. Value of FDG PET imaging in the management of patients with thyroid, neuroendocrine, and neural crest tumors. Clin Nucl Med 2004;29:86–90.

65. Sundin A, Eriksson B, Bergstrom M, et al. PET in the diagnosis of neuroendocrine tumors. Ann N Y Acad Sci 2004;1014:246–57.

66. Zhao DS, Valdivia AY, Li Y, et al. 18F-fluorodeoxyglucose positron emission tomography in small-cell lung cancer. Semin Nucl Med 2002;32:272–5.

67. Diehl M, Risse JH, Brandt-Mainz K, et al. Fluorine-18 fluorodeoxyglucose positron emission tomography in medullary thyroid cancer: results of a multicentre study. Eur J Nucl Med 2001;28:1671–6.

68. Shulkin BL, Wieland DM, Baro ME, et al. PET hydroxyephedrine imaging of neuroblastoma. J Nucl Med 1996;37:16–21.

69. Shulkin BL, Wieland DM, Schwaiger M, et al. PET scanning with hydroxyephedrine: an approach to the localization of pheochromocytoma. J Nucl Med 1992;33:1125–31.

70. Abbruzzese JL, Abbruzzese MC, Lenzi R, et al. Analysis of a diagnostic strategy for patients with suspected tumors of unknown origin. J Clin Oncol 1995;13:2094–103.

71. Didolkar MS, Fanous N, Elias EG, et al. Metastatic carcinomas from occult primary tumors: a study of 254 patients. Ann Surg 1977;186:625–30.

72. Le Chevalier T, Cvitkovic E, Caille P, et al. Early metastatic cancer of unknown primary origin at presentation: a clinical study of 302 consecutive autopsied patients. Arch Intern Med 1988;148:2035–9.

73. Steckel RJ, Kagan AR. Diagnostic persistence in working up metastatic cancer with an unknown primary site. Radiology 1980;134:367–9.

74. Naresh KN. Do metastatic tumours from an unknown primary reflect angiogenic incompetence of the tumour at the primary site? A hypothesis. Med Hypotheses 2002;59:357–60.

75. Raber MN, Faintuch J, Abbruzzese JL, et al. Continuous infusion 5-fluorouracil, etoposide and cis-diamminedichloroplatinum in patients with metastatic carcinoma of unknown primary origin. Ann Oncol 1991;2:519–20.

76. Alberini JL, Belhocine T, Hustinx R, et al. Whole-body positron emission tomography using fluorodeoxyglucose in patients with metastases of unknown primary tumours (CUP syndrome). Nucl Med Commun 2003;24:1081–6.

77. Bohuslavizki KH, Klutmann S, Kroger S, et al. FDG PET detection of unknown primary tumors. J Nucl Med 2000;41:816–22.

78. Freudenberg LS, Fischer M, Antoch G, et al. Dual modality of 18F-fluorodeoxyglucose-positron emission tomography/computed tomography in patients with cervical carcinoma of unknown primary. Med Princ Pract 2005;14:155–60.

79. Gutzeit A, Antoch G, Kuhl H, et al. Unknown primary tumors: detection with dual-modality PFT/CT: initial experience. Radiology 2005;234:227–34.

80. Kole AC, Nieweg OE, Pruim J, et al. Detection of unknown occult primary tumors using positron emission tomography. Cancer 1998;82:1160–6.

81. Syed R, Bomanji JB, Nagabhushan N, et al. Impact of combined (18)F-FDG PET/CT in head and neck tumours. Br J Cancer 2005;92:1046–50.

82. Ambrosini V, Tomassetti P, Rubello D, et al. Role of 18F-dopa PET/CT imaging in the management of patients with 111In-pentetreotide negative GEP tumours. Nucl Med Commun 2007;28:473–7.

83. Pasquali C, Sperti C, Scappin S, et al. Role and indications of fluorodeoxyglucose positron emission tomography (FDG-PET) in neuroendocrine pancreatico-duodenal tumors. J pancreas 2004;6 (5 Suppl):528–9.

84. Oh SW, Prasad V, Lee DS, et al. Monitoring response to peptide receptor radionuclide therapy (PRRT) in patients with metastasised neuroendocrine tumours (NET): intraindividual comparison between Ga-68-DOTA-NOC, F-18-FDG-PET/CT, and CT alone [abstract EPOS]. European Society of Radiology Conference. Vienna, March 7-11, 2008.

Positron Emission Tomography Imaging and Hyperinsulinism

Miguel Hernandez-Pampaloni, MD, PhD[a],
Hongming Zhuang, MD, PhD[b], Stefano Fanti, MD[c],
Abass Alavi, MD, PhD[a],*

KEYWORDS

- Positron emission tomography
- Fluorodopa • Hyperinsulinism • Pediatrics

Congenital hyperinsulinism (HI), formerly termed nesidioblastosis, is the most common cause of persistent hypoglycemia in infants and children.[1] Infants with severe forms of this disorder present with hypoglycemia in the newborn period and require glucose infusion at rates as high as 20 mg/kg to 30 mg/kg per minute to control blood glucose levels. The importance of early diagnosis of HI cannot be overemphasized because persistent, dangerously low blood glucose levels can lead to disorders, such as seizures and permanent brain damage, which occur in up to 20% of patients with the severe form of this disorder.[2,3] Mutations in at least five genes have been associated with congenital hyperinsulinism. They encode glucokinase, glutamate dehydrogenase, the mitochondrial enzyme short-chain 3-hydroxyacyl-CoA dehydrogenase, and the two components (sulfonylurea receptor 1 and potassium inward rectifying channel, subfamily J, member 11) of the adenosine triphosphate (ATP)-sensitive potassium (K) channels (K_{ATP} channels). K_{ATP} hyperinsulinism is the most common and severe form of congenital hyperinsulinism. In recent years, it has become clear that the failure of regulation of insulin release in HI has different causes, including abnormalities in ABCC8 and KCNJ11 genes, which encode the sulfonylurea receptor 1 (SUR1) and Kir6.2 subunits of a β-cell ATP-sensitive potassium channel K_{ATP}[4,5] and mutations of the genes for glucokinase (GK, MIM.138079),[6] for glutamate dehydrogenase (GLUD1, MIM.138130).[7]

PATHOGENESIS AND CLINICAL COURSE

HI typically presents in the first few days after birth for term and preterm infants with symptomatic hypoglycemia.[8] The patients may present with nonspecific symptoms of hypoglycemia, such as poor feeding, lethargy, and irritability, or with neurologic symptoms, such as seizures and coma. However, subtle forms of HI may present later in infancy or even childhood. Hypoglycemia is usually persistent and normoglycemia can only be achieved by administering concentrated intravenous dextrose infusions. A blood sample taken at the time of hypoglycemia will show inappropriately elevated serum insulin levels, with low serum fatty acid concentrations and ketone bodies.[9] This unregulated insulin secretion increases the glucose consumption by insulin-sensitive tissues, such as muscle, adipose tissue, and liver, while simultaneously suppressing hepatic glucose production (both glycogenolysis and gluconeogenesis), lipolysis, and ketogenesis. The serum lactate level may be elevated in some forms of HI and the serum

[a] Department of Radiology, Hospital of the University of Pennsylvania, 3470 Spruce Street, Philadelphia, PA 19104, USA
[b] Department of Radiology, Children's Hospital of Philadelphia, Philadelphia, PA 19104, USA
[c] Department of Nuclear Medicine, S Orsola Hospital, Bologna, Italy
* Corresponding author.
E-mail address: abass.alavi@uphs.upenn.edu (A. Alavi).

PET Clin 2 (2008) 377–383
doi:10.1016/j.cpet.2008.05.003

ammonia concentration must be measured in all patients presenting with HI because of the association with hyperinsulinism/hyperammonemia syndrome.[7]

Patients with HI usually undergo a trial of medical therapy with diazoxide, glucagon, octreotide, or continuous feedings to control hypoglycemia. However, a significant number of patients will fail to respond to this regimen and will require surgical intervention. Although two histologically and genetically distinct groups are now recognized among patients with K_{ATP} defects, diffuse and focal HI[10], there are still some cases which represent a diagnostic challenge, as they cannot be easily classified into either group.[11] Even though diffuse and focal forms share a similar clinical presentation, they result from different pathphysiologic and molecular mechanisms. The typical diffuse form affects all the β-cells and is most commonly caused by recessive mutations in the genes encoding the two subunits of the K_{ATP} channel. The focal form (focal adenomatous pancreatic hyperplasia) of HI is found in about 40% to 50% of the children and appears to be localized to one region of the pancreas.

In general, patients who are homozygous or compound heterozygous for ABCC8 or KCNJ11 recessive mutations have diffuse HI, and they show enlargement of islet cell nuclei throughout the pancreas. These patients usually require near total pancreatectomy (95%–98% resection) to achieve manageable control of blood sugar levels. However, with near total pancreatectomy, there is a high risk of diabetes immediately after surgery or later in life.[12] In contrast, focal HI is caused by a paternally inherited K_{ATP} mutation together with a somatic loss of heterozygosity for the maternal 11p gene.[13] Resection of the adenomatous focus has a potential to cure patients with focal disease if the remaining pancreas is kept intact.[14]

DIAGNOSTIC METHODS

The current standard method for differentiating between the focal and diffuse forms of the disease consists of intraoperative histologic examination of multiple tissue samples as frozen sections. This method requires considerable expertise (surgical and histopathologic) and can be reliably performed only in selected institutions.[11,15] Because focal HI is a potentially curable disorder, attempts have been made to establish this diagnosis before surgery. Conventional imaging methods, such as ultrasound, computed tomography, and magnetic resonance imaging have proven of no value for this purpose. As a result, interventional radiologic methods have been commonly used for locating focal lesions. Transhepatic portal venous sampling (THPVS) has been employed with only a modest degree of success.[16,17] This method relies upon transhepatic catheterization of the draining veins and demonstration of persistent insulin secretion in spite of a low blood glucose concentration from one or more anatomic sites in the pancreas. However, this technique is technically difficult to perform and requires stopping all medications for at least 48 hours before the procedure, which may expose the infant to a prolonged period of hypoglycemia.

Selective intra-arterial calcium stimulation of the pancreas with hepatic venous sampling (ASVS) is another method that has been demonstrated to show markedly elevated baseline insulin levels throughout the pancreas of the infants with diffuse HI. This invasive procedure does not reliably distinguish patients with focal HI from those with diffuse disease[18–20] ASVS has about the same degree of accuracy as THPVS in correctly identifying the region of focal lesions in only 70% of cases. Selective intra-arterial calcium stimulation is associated with significant risks during general anesthesia, endotracheal intubation, and femoral artery catheterization, and also results in substantial levels of radiation exposure. In addition, blood transfusion is frequently required to maintain normal blood volume following multiple sampling for the required analyses. It should be noted that both THPVS and ASVS are associated with dangerous levels of radiation exposure, which are becoming a source of concern for developing certain malignancies in the pediatric population. Therefore, routine use of these procedures is unjustified.

SPECT IMAGING

Receptors for somatostatin have been identified on many cells of neuroendocrine origin.[21] Scintigraphy with radiolabeled somatostatin analogs using 111Indium-DTPA-octreotide has been shown to have high accuracy for visualization of neuroendocrine tumors.[22,23] When compared with conventional imaging modalities, such as computed tomography, magnetic resonance imaging, and ultrasound for detecting primary and metastatic gastrinomas, somatostatin receptor scintigraphy was found to be the single most sensitive imaging method for detecting this tumor.[24] Somatostatin receptor scintigraphy changes the surgical therapeutic strategy in up to 25% of the patients with neuroendocrine tumors.[25] Importantly, the findings by somatostatin receptor scintigraphy of receptor-positive tumors can predict a beneficial effect from appropriate therapies with radiolabeled octreotide.[26] However, the spatial resolution of somatostatin receptor scintigraphy with indium-111 octreotide is markedly inferior when compared with computed tomography or magnetic resonance imaging.

POSITRON EMISSION TOMOGRAPHY

Positron emission tomography (PET) has overcome many of the shortcomings that are encountered with conventional imaging techniques.[27] The critical role of PET imaging with fluorodeoxyglucose (FDG) and certain other tracers in the management of a number of serious disorders, especially in the fields of oncology, neurology and cardiology, has been well established. Unfortunately, FDG-PET has been of limited value for assessing neuroendocrine tumors. Tumors with high proliferative activity and poor differentiation have been shown to have an increased FDG uptake.[28] This has been noted by several studies which have demonstrated that FDG is taken up in most tumors with clinicopathologically aggressive neuroendocrine tumors, while only a minority of patients with slow growing tumors showed a slightly increased FDG accumulation.[29] Another study failed to visualize carcinoid tumors by FDG-PET.[30]

Neuroendocrine cells have the capacity to take up decarboxylate amine precursors, such as L-dihydroxyphenylalanine (L-DOPA) and 5-hydroxy-1-tryptophan (5-HTP), and to store their biogenic amines.[31,32] The re-uptake of monoamines most likely proceeds via selective sodium/chloride dependent monoamine transporters of the plasma membrane.[33,34] Amine precursors, such as 5-HTP and L-DOPA, thus may be taken up by the tumor cells and through the action of aromatic amino acid decarboxylase (AADC). These precursors become decarboxylated and are converted to the corresponding amines dopamine and serotonin. Accumulation of monoamines into secretory vesicles within the cytoplasm is achieved by vesicular monoamine transporters.[35] In response to specific stimuli, they translocate to the cell membrane and their content is released into circulation through exocytosis.

L-DOPA is a catecholamine precursor that is converted to dopamine by the aromatic AADC. Based on its known biochemical pathway and the prior experience with regard to imaging of the dopaminergic system in the brain, amine precursor L-DOPA has been considered a potential candidate to examine endocrine tumors. The first synthesis of 5-[18F]fluoro-DOPA was reported by Firnau and colleagues[36] in 1973. Because of the proximity of the fluorine atom to the hydroxyl groups of FDOPA, 6-[18F]fluoro-L-DOPA was developed and the first FDOPA-PET brain study was performed in 1983 to visualize the dopaminergic neurons in the basal ganglia.[37] As a neurotransmitter substance in the central and peripheral nervous system, FDOPA has been successfully used to assess patients with movement disorders, including Parkinson's disease. Patients with early Parkinson's disease have reduced accumulation of this tracer in the putamen contralateral to the affected limb, with relative sparing of the caudate.[38] Significant correlations between FDOPA uptake and motor symptoms have also been reported.[39]

Pancreatic cells contain markers associated with neuroendocrine cells, such as tyrosine hydroxylase, dopamine, neuronal dopamine transporter, vesicular dopamine transporter, and monoamine oxidase A and B. Pancreatic islets have been shown to take up L-DOPA and convert it to dopamine through the AADC.[40] Initially L-DOPA labeled with 11C and PET imaging were used to study patients with pancreatic endocrine tumors.[41] When compared with conventional computed tomography, only 50% of the tumors were visualized with this technique, but nonfunctioning tumors and small insulinomas were undetectable. Since the publication of this original article, FDOPA-PET imaging has been reported to provide a higher sensitivity when compared with conventional techniques and, therefore, may potentially alter patient management in about one third of patients with gastrointestinal carcinoid tumors.[42,43] In addition, FDOPA has been successfully tested in medullary thyroid carcinoma and pheochromocytoma for staging lymph node metastasis.[44-47]

During recent years, by using FDOPA and modern PET cameras, promising preliminary data have been reported for distinguishing between focal and diffuse forms of HI. After a fasting period of 6 hours and having discontinued medications for at least 72 hours, Otonkoski and colleagues[48] and Ribeiro and colleagues[49] studied a group of 15 neonates with a clinical diagnosis of HI. Focal uptake of FDOPA was seen in five patients while diffuse activity was noted in the remaining patients. All patients with focal and four with diffuse uptake underwent surgical intervention and histologic examination, which confirmed the PET scan findings. Barthlen and colleagues[50] and Kauhanen and colleagues[51] have reported similar results in limited samples, suggesting the value of this noninvasive imaging modality in precisely diagnosing focal forms of HI. Recent investigations reported that immunohistochemical detection of DOPA decarboxylase showed diffuse staining of Langerhans islets in the whole pancreas in patients with diffuse HI. In contrast, dense focal staining was

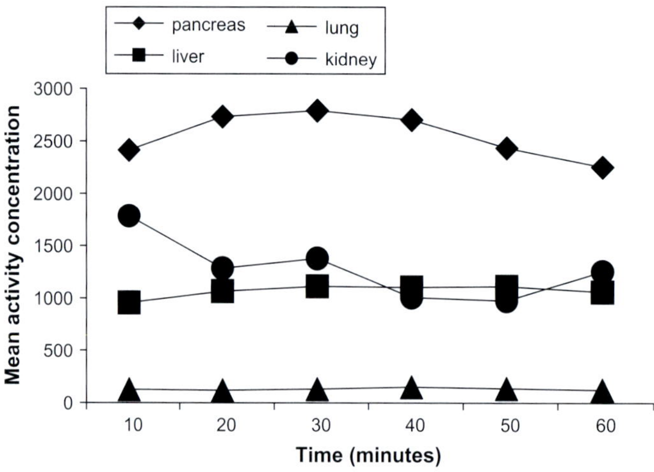

Fig. 1. Counts distribution of FDOPA along the 60-minute acquisition in the pancreas, compared with surrounding organs, in a patient with focal HI disease.

seen in patients with focal disease. These results reinforce the notion that FDOPA can selectively depict diverse molecular pancreatic pathophysiologic mechanisms.[52]

The largest data generated by using FDOPA-PET imaging in the HI patient have been reported following a joint effort between the Hospital of the University of Pennsylvania and the Hyperinsulinism Center of the Children's Hospital of Philadelphia. After the first preliminary data were published, Hardy and colleagues[53,54] studied 50 infants with HI unresponsive to medical therapy. Following the intravenous administration of 3 MBq/kg to 6 MBq/kg of [18F]-DOPA, dynamic PET images were obtained for 50 to 60 minutes. Distribution of FDOPA remained constant during the acquisition time, with minimal uptake in the surrounding organs (with the exception of the physiologic renal excretion), providing an excellent target-to-background ratio (**Figs. 1** and **2**). Images

were routinely coregistered with the contrast-enhanced computed tomography scans of the abdomen in these children. All surgical interventions were performed by the same surgeon, using careful palpation and inspection of the pancreas to identify focal lesions. An example of a patient with pancreatic focal disease in the head of the pancreas is depicted in **Fig. 3**. On the other hand, the characteristic uniform uptake along the entire pancreas is noted in a patient with the diffuse form of HI in **Fig. 4**.

After comparing the PET scan interpretations with histologic diagnoses from intraoperative frozen section biopsies, the investigators reported an accuracy of 88% for differentiating between focal or diffuse HI. FDOPA PET accurately diagnosed 75% of all focal cases and had a 100% accuracy for identifying the location of the lesion within the pancreas. Because of the high accuracy of FDOPA PET in localizing these lesions, this

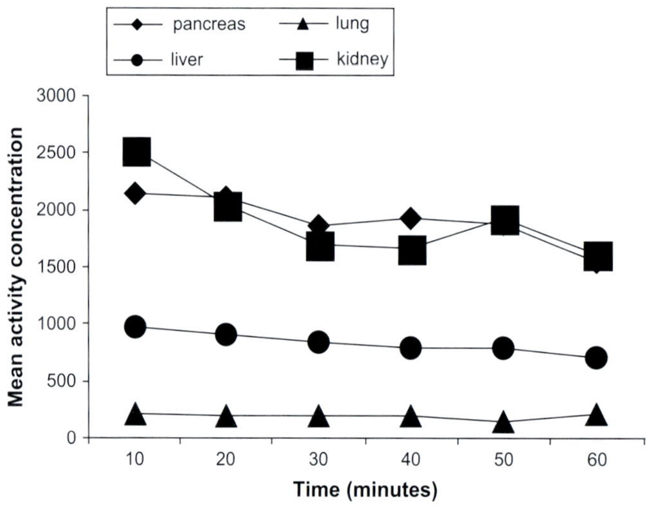

Fig. 2. Counts distribution of FDOPA along the 60-minute acquisition in the pancreas, compared with surrounding organs, in a patient with diffuse HI disease.

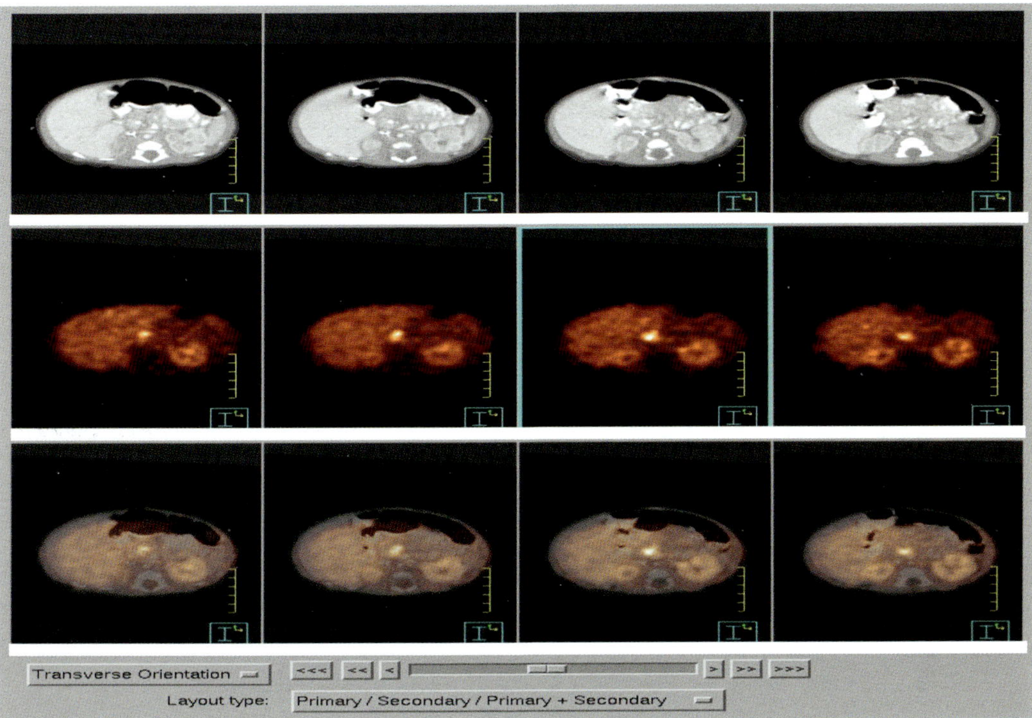

Fig. 3. Axial images of abdominal computed tomography, FDOPA PET, and coregistered PET/CT in a patient with focal disease.

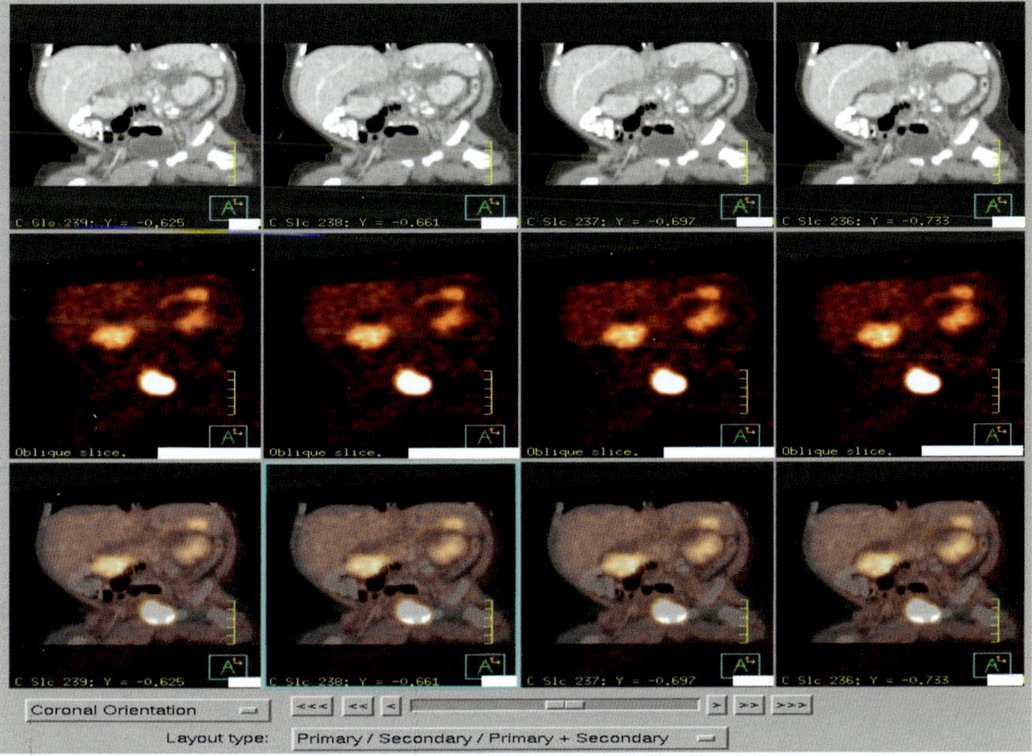

Fig. 4. Axial images of abdominal computed tomography, FDOPA PET, and coregistered PET/CT in a patient with focal disease.

imaging technique can be used as a standard procedure for managing patients who are afflicted with a medically untreatable form of HI.

These data demonstrate the crucial clinical benefit of noninvasive FDOPA-PET imaging for identifying focal and diffuse forms of HI, and it opens the door for other potential applications of this compound in the field. This imaging technique may prove to be useful in the future understanding of the mechanisms of pancreatic insulin regulation, and may be applied to more common metabolic diseases, such as diabetes. The method could potentially be of value in monitoring patients with beta (islet) cell transplantation as well.

REFERENCES

1. Stanley CA. Hyperinsulinism in infants and children. Pediatr Clin North Am 1997;44(2):363–74.
2. Meissner T, Brune W, Mayatepek E. Persistent hyperinsulinaemic hypoglycaemia of infancy: therapy, clinical outcome and mutational analysis. Eur J Pediatr 1997;156(10):754–7.
3. Menni F, de Lonlay P, Sevin C, et al. Neurologic outcomes of 90 neonates and infants with persistent hyperinsulinemic hypoglycemia. Pediatrics 2001; 107(3):476–9.
4. Thomas P, Ye Y, Lightner E. Mutation of the pancreatic islet inward rectifier Kir6.2 also leads to familial persistent hyperinsulinemic hypoglycemia of infancy. Hum Mol Genet 1996;5(11):1809–12.
5. Nestorowicz A, Inagaki N, Gonoi T, et al. A nonsense mutation in the inward rectifier potassium channel gene, Kir6.2, is associated with familial hyperinsulinism. Diabetes 1997;46(11):1743–8.
6. Glaser B, Kesavan P, Heyman M, et al. Familial hyperinsulinism caused by an activating glucokinase mutation. N Engl J Med 1998;338(4):226–30.
7. Stanley CA, Lieu YK, Hsu BY, et al. Hyperinsulinism and hyperammonemia in infants with regulatory mutations of the glutamate dehydrogenase gene. N Engl J Med 1998;338(19):1352–7.
8. Hussain K, Aynsley-Green A. Hyperinsulinemic hypoglycaemia in preterm neonates. Arch Dis Child Fetal Neonatal Ed 2004;89:F65–7.
9. Aynsley-Green A, Hussain K, Hall J, et al. Practical management of hyperinsulinism in infancy. Arch Dis Child Fetal Neonatal Ed 2000;82:F98–107.
10. Sempoux C, Guiot Y, Lefevre A, et al. Neonatal hyperinsulinemic hypoglycemia: heterogeneity of the syndrome and keys for differential diagnosis. J Clin Endocrinol Metab 1998;83(5):1455–61.
11. Suchi M, MacMullen C, Thornton PS, et al. Histopathology of congenital hyperinsulinism: retrospective study with genotype correlations. Pediatr Dev Pathol 2003;6:322–33.
12. Shilyansky J, Fisher S, Cutz E, et al. Is 95% pancreatectomy the procedure of choice for treatment of persistent hyperinsulinemic hypoglycemia of the neonate? J Pediatr Surg 1997;32(2):342–6.
13. Verkarre V, Fournet JC, de Lonlay P, et al. Paternal mutation of the sulfonylurea receptor (SUR1) gene and maternal loss of 11p15 imprinted genes lead to persistent hyperinsulinism in focal adenomatous hyperplasia. J Clin Invest 1998;102(7):1286–91.
14. de Lonlay-Debeney P, Poggi-Travert F, et al. Clinical features of 52 neonates with hyperinsulinism. N Engl J Med 1999;340(15):1169–75.
15. Rahier J, Sempoux C, Fournet JC, et al. Partial or near-total pancreatectomy for persistent neonatal hyperinsulinaemic hypoglycaemia: the pathologist's role. Histopathology 1998;32(1):15–9.
16. Dubois J, Brunelle F, Touati G, et al. Hyperinsulinism in children: diagnostic value of pancreatic venous sampling correlated with clinical, pathological and surgical outcome in 25 cases. Pediatr Radiol 1995; 25(7):512–6.
17. Fekete CN, de Lonlay P, Jaubert F, et al. The surgical management of congenital hyperinsulinemic hypoglycemia in infancy. J Pediatr Surg 2004;39(3):267–9.
18. Ferry RJ Jr, Kelly A, Grimberg A, et al. Calcium-stimulated insulin secretion in diffuse and focal forms of congenital hyperinsulinism. J Pediatr 2000;137(2):239–46.
19. Stanley CA, Thornton PS, Ganguly A, et al. Preoperative evaluation of infants with focal or diffuse congenital hyperinsulinism by intravenous acute insulin response tests and selective pancreatic arterial calcium stimulation. J Clin Endocrinol Metab 2004;89(1):288–96.
20. Grimberg A, Ferry RJ Jr, Kelly A, et al. Dysregulation of insulin secretion in children with congenital hyperinsulinism due to sulfonylurea receptor mutations. Diabetes 2001;50(2):322–8.
21. Patel YC, Amherdt M, Orci L, et al. Quantitative electron microscopic autoradiography of insulin, glucagon, and somatostatin binding sites on islets. Science 1982;217(4565):1155–6.
22. Krenning EP, Bakker WH, Kooij PP, et al. Somatostatin receptor scintigraphy with indium-111-DTPA-D-Phe-1-octreotide in man: metabolism, dosimetry and comparison with iodine-123-Tyr-3-octreotide. J Nucl Med 1992;33(5):652–8.
23. Kwekkeboom DJ, Krenning EP, Bakker WH, et al. Somatostatin analogue scintigraphy in carcinoid tumours. Eur J Nucl Med 1993;20(4):283–92.
24. Gibril F, Reynolds JC, Doppman JL, et al. Somatostatin receptor scintigraphy: its sensitivity compared with that of other imaging methods in detecting primary and metastatic gastrinomas. A prospective study. Ann Intern Med 1996;125(1):26–34.
25. Lebtahi R, Cadiot G, Sarda L, et al. Clinical impact of somatostatin receptor scintigraphy in the management of patients with neuroendocrine

gastroenteropancreatic tumors. J Nucl Med 1997; 38(6):853–8.

26. Janson ET, Westlin JE, Eriksson B, et al. [111In-DTPA-D-Phe1]octreotide scintigraphy in patients with carcinoid tumours: the predictive value for somatostatin analogue treatment. Eur J Endocrinol 1994;131(6):577–81.

27. Alavi A, Lakhani P, Mavi A, et al. PET: a revolution in medical imaging. Radiol Clin North Am 2004;42(6): 983–1001, vii.

28. Adams S, Baum R, Hertel A, et al. Limited value of fluorine-18 fluorodeoxyglucose positron emission tomography for the imaging of neuroendocrine tumours. Eur J Nucl Med 1998;25(1):79–83.

29. Pasquali C, Rubello D, Sperti C, et al. Neuroendocrine tumor imaging: can 18F-fluorodeoxyglucose positron emission tomography detect tumors with poor prognosis and aggressive behavior? World J Surg 1998;22(6):588–92.

30. Jadvar H, Segall GM. False-negative fluorine-18-FDG PET in metastatic carcinoid. J Nucl Med 1997;38(9):1382–3.

31. Baylin SB, Abeloff MD, Goodwin G, et al. Activities of L-dopa decarboxylase and diamine oxidase (histaminase) in human lung cancers and decarboxylase as a marker for small (oat) cell cancer in cell culture. Cancer Res 1980;40(6):1990–4.

32. Berger CL, de Bustros A, Roos BA, et al. Human medullary thyroid carcinoma in culture provides a model relating growth dynamics, endocrine cell differentiation, and tumor progression. J Clin Endocrinol Metab 1984;59(2):338–43.

33. Shimada S, Kitayama S, Lin CL, et al. Cloning and expression of a cocaine-sensitive dopamine transporter complementary DNA. Science 1991; 254(5031):576–8.

34. Giros B, el Mestikawy S, Godinot N, et al. Cloning, pharmacological characterization, and chromosome assignment of the human dopamine transporter. Mol Pharmacol 1992;42(3):383–90.

35. Holtje M, von Jagow B, Pahner I, et al. The neuronal monoamine transporter VMAT2 is regulated by the trimeric GTPase Go(2). J Neurosci 2000;20(6):2131–41.

36. Firnau G, Nahmias C, Garnett ES. The preparation of [18F]5-fluoro-DOPA with reactor produced fluorine-18. Int J Appl Radiat Isot 1973;24:182–4.

37. Garnett ES, Firnau G, Nahmias C. Dopamine visualized in the basal ganglia of living man. Nature 1983; 305:137–8.

38. Nahmias C, Garnett ES, Firnau G, et al. Striatal dopamine distribution in Parkinsonian patients during life. J Neurol Sci 1985;69(3):223–30.

39. Reichmann H. Neuroprotection in idiopathic Parkinson's disease. J Neurol 2002;249(Suppl 3):III21–3.

40. Lindstrom P. Aromatic-L-amino-acid decarboxylase activity in mouse pancreatic islets. Biochim Biophys Acta 1986;884(2):276–81.

41. Ahlstrom H, Eriksson B, Bergstrom M, et al. Pancreatic neuroendocrine tumors: diagnosis with PET. Radiology 1995;195(2):333–7.

42. Hoegerle S, Altehoefer C, Ghanem M, et al. Whole-body 18F dopa PET for detection of gastrointestinal carcinoid tumors. Radiology 2001;220(2):373–80.

43. Becherer A, Szabo M, Karanikas G, et al. Imaging of advanced neuroendocrine tumors with (18)F-FDOPA PET. J Nucl Med 2004;45(7):1161–7.

44. Hoegerle S, Altehoefer C, Ghanem M, et al. 18FDOPA positron emission tomography for tumour detection in patients with medullary thyroid carcinoma and elevated calcitonin levels. Eur J Nucl Med 2001; 28(1):64–71.

45. Hoegerle S, Nitzsche E, Altehoefer C, et al. Pheochromocytomas: detection with 18F DOPA whole body PET–initial results. Radiology 2002;222(2):507–12.

46. Ilias I, Yu J, Carrasquillo JA, et al. Superiority of 6-[18F]-fluorodopamine positron emission tomography versus [131I]-metaiodobenzylguanidine scintigraphy in the localization of metastatic pheochromocytoma. J Clin Endocrinol Metab 2003;88(9):4083–7.

47. Pacak K, Eisenhofer G, Golstein DS, et al. Functional imaging of endocrine tumors: role of positron emission tomography. Endocr Rev 2004;25(4):568–80.

48. Otonkoski T, Nanto-Salonen K, Seppanen M, et al. Noninvasive diagnosis of focal hyperinsulinism of infancy with [18F]-DOPA positron emission tomography. Diabetes 2006;55:13–8.

49. Ribeiro MJ, De Lonlay P, Delzescaux T, et al. Characterization of hyperinsulinism in infancy assessed with PET and 18F-fluoro-L-DOPA. J Nucl Med 2005;46:5460–566.

50. Barthlen W, Blankenstein O, Mau H, et al. Evaluation of (18F) FDOPA PET-CT for surgery in focal congenital hyperinsulinism. J Clin Endocrinol Metab 2008; 93(3):869–75.

51. Kauhanen S, Seppanen M, Minn H, et al. Fluorine-18-L-dihydroxyphenylalanine (18F-DOPA) positron emission tomography as a tool to localize an insulinoma or beta-cell hyperplasia in adult patients. J Clin Endocrinol Metab 2007;92(4):1237–44.

52. de Lonlay P, Simon-Carre A, Ribeiro MJ. Congenital hyperinsulinism: pancreatic [18F]fluoro-L-dihydroxyphenylalanine (DOPA) positron emission tomography and immunohistochemistry study of DOPA decarboxylase and insulin secretion. J Clin Endocrinol Metab 2006;91(3):933–40.

53. Hardy OT, Hernandez-Pampaloni M, Saffer JR, et al. Diagnosis and localization of focal congenital hyperinsulinism by 18F-fluorodopa PET scan. J Pediatr 2007;150:140–5.

54. Hardy OT, Hernandez-Pampaloni M, Saffer JR. Accuracy of [18F]fluorodopa positron emission tomography for diagnosing and localizing focal congenital hyperinsulinism. J Clin Endocrinol Metab 2007;92: 4706–11.

PET and Parathyroid

Gaia Grassetto, MD[a], Abass Alavi, MD, PhD[b],
Domenico Rubello, MD[a],*

KEYWORDS

- Hyperparathyroidism • 99mTc-Sestamibi
- PET/CT imaging • 11C-methionine

Conventional nuclear medicine plays an important role in the detection and diagnosis of parathyroid disease, especially primary hyperparathyroidism. It is widely used for this purpose by administering technetium-labeled compounds. Parathyroid scintigraphy with sestamibi is particularly useful in confirming the diagnosis of hyperparathyroidism, localizing the pathologic gland, and selecting the patients in whom a minimally invasive surgical treatment can be offered an appropriate approach. The purpose of this article is to describe the currently available and potential new techniques along with the benefits and limitations of several acquisition protocols. We also describe the possible use of PET in parathyroid disease, with its high spatial and contrast resolutions and its ability for precise anatomic localization of the involved sites. Currently, the use of positron emission tomography (PET) in this disease is still limited, and a clear clinical role for this powerful imaging modality has not yet been completely defined. This is likely due, at least in part, to the availability of effective conventional imaging techniques, such as sestamibi planar and single photon emission CT (SPECT) imaging techniques. These imaging techniques have been reported to have sensitivity and accuracy approaching 90% in primary hyperparathyroidism. There is still a group of patients who have hyperparathyroidism in whom making a diagnosis of enlarged parathyroids remains difficult, however, especially patients who have secondary and tertiary hyperparathyroidism. In these cases PET and CT with novel radiopharmaceuticals are expected to play an important role.

ANATOMIC AND PHYSIOLOGIC CONSIDERATIONS

Parathyroid glands originate from pharyngeal pouches and generally are in groups of four, but occasionally they may appear numerous (2%–5% of population).[1,2] They are usually localized behind the thyroid gland: two behind the upper lobe (originating from the fourth pouch) and two behind the lower lobe (originating from the third pouch).[1,2] The location of normal inferior parathyroid glands, however, is variable, probably because of the variable migration process. They can be intrathyroidal or within the thyrothymic ligament, the thymus, or the mediastinum. The accessory glands have various locations from the cricoid cartilage up to the lower mediastinum and are derived from the numerous dorsal and ventral wings of the pouches.[1] The normal glands differ considerably in shape and size between individuals and within the same individual. Usually they are ovoid or bean-shaped and weigh approximately 30 to 40 mg each.[1]

The parathyroid gland has two main components: parenchymal cells and fat cells. The number of fat cells varies with age; the number is small until adolescence and then increases gradually and constitutes 10% to 25% of glandular volume by 30 years of age.[1] In a normal gland, parenchymal cells are predominantly chief cells, the active endocrine cells that produce parathyroid hormone (PTH). Oxyphilic and transitional-oxyphilic cells noted in this gland increase with age and that may produce PTH. In addition to these parenchymal and fat cells, there are clear cells that have no known function and are thought to be fundamentally inactive.[1]

a Department of Nuclear Medicine, PET Center, 'S. Maria della Misercordia' Rovigo Hospital, Istituto Oncologico Veneto (IOV)-IRCCS, Viale Tre Martiri 140, 45100 Rovigo, Italy
b Division of Nuclear Medicine, Hospital of the University of Pennsylvania, University of Pennsylvania School of Medicine, Philadelphia, PA, USA
* Corresponding author.
E-mail address: domenico.rubello@libero.it (D. Rubello).

PET Clin 2 (2008) 385–393
doi:10.1016/j.cpet.2008.04.005

The major factor for PTH secretion is the blood ionized calcium level because its reduction stimulates PTH production and secretion. PTH is responsible for maintaining calcium homeostasis, which it does in four ways: (1) by causing increased calcium absorption from gastrointestinal tract, (2) by stimulating osteoclastic activity, which results in reabsorption of calcium and phosphate from bone, (3) by inhibiting phosphate reabsorption by the proximal renal tubules, and (4) by enhancing renal tubular calcium reabsorption.[1,2]

HYPERPARATHYROIDISM

Hyperparathyroidism is a condition of increased production and secretion of PTH. It may exist as a primary, secondary, or tertiary disease.[1] Primary hyperparathyroidism is most common and is caused by adenomatous or hyperplastic changes in the parathyroid glands. It has been associated with a carcinomatous parathyroid gland or a nonparathyroidal tumor, such as a bronchogenic tumor or renal cell carcinoma that ectopically secretes PTH or a biologically similar product. The latter causes are rare. Approximately 80% of patients with primary hyperparathyroidism have a solitary adenoma, a benign tumor mainly formed by chief cells, with a weight that can vary from 100 mg to more than 100 mg. The size generally correlates with the degree of hypercalcemia.[1] Hyperplasia of the parathyroid glands occurs in less than 20% of patients, whereas carcinoma is rare and occurs in less than 1% of patients.[1]

Secondary hyperparathyroidism is generally caused by chronic hypocalcemia, such as renal failure, malabsorption conditions, dietary rickets, or ingestion of drugs that decrease intestinal absorption of calcium (ie, phenytoin, phenobarbital, laxatives). Secondary hyperparathyroidism is solely a compensatory hyperplasia of the parathyroid glands in response to hypocalcemia.[1] Tertiary hyperparathyroidism is a condition in which parathyroid hyperplasia, consequent to chronic hypocalcemia, becomes autonomous with development of hypercalcemia. These pathologic reactionary conditions do not regress after the correction of the cause of hypocalcemia.[1]

In recent years, hyperparathyroidism has been diagnosed with increased frequency because of advanced laboratory tests that allow detection of subtle disease on a routine chemistry screening panel. The diagnosis of hyperparathyroidism is becoming a common observation in which it is detected in the subclinical states, and as such this disease is noted without complications such as nephrocalcinosis, urolithiasis, bone disease, and neuropsychiatric disturbances.[1]

DIAGNOSTIC IMAGING

In the past, many surgeons would operate on patients with primary hyperparathyroidism without the use of preoperative localization imaging. In 1986, Doppman stated that the best way to localize the diseased parathyroid gland is to locate an experienced surgeon.[3] In contrast, in cases of recurrent disease after surgery, the use of preoperative imaging is mandatory and widely accepted. The recent development of minimally invasive surgery of the neck (endoscopic, video-assisted, and radio-guided) has led to increased interest in the use of preoperative localization imaging in cases of primary hyperthyroidism and in patients with recurrent disease.[4–8]

There are various imaging techniques for this purpose, but no ideal method consistently provides high sensitivity and specificity for all cases. Structural imaging, such as CT, ultrasonography (US), and MR imaging, cannot always distinguish between functional parathyroid tissue and unrelated findings. They do, however, provide excellent image resolution and good contrast. Their reported percentages of success vary from 36% to 75%.[5,9–13] Functional imaging in general and technetium 99m Tc-sestamibi parathyroid scintigraphy in particular have a sensitivity value that reaches 90% or more.[14] The specificity is low, especially in the presence of nodular thyroid goiter,[1,7,15] but it can be improved by using scintigraphy with a dual-tracer protocol (imaging thyroid with iodide 123 I iodide and technetium 99m Tc-sestamibi) and subtraction imaging.[14] Use of tomographic imaging (SPECT) of the neck and thorax, especially in patients with recurrent hyperparathyroidism after prior surgery, is also useful. To further improve specificity, combined parathyroid sestamibi scintigraphy and structural imaging of the neck, in particular high-resolution US, has proved to be of value.

Currently, there is a general agreement that PET is most useful in cases in which US and sestamibi scintigraphy have failed, most often in secondary and tertiary hyperparathyroidism (generally in patients with renal failure on chronic hemodialysis).[16]

Conventional Nuclear Medicine Imaging: Sestamibi

In the late 1980s, by chance during myocardial perfusion studies, Coakley and colleagues observed significant uptake of technetium 99m Tc-sestamibi in abnormal parathyroid tissue of patients with primary hyperparathyroidism. As a result, parathyroid scintigraphy with sestamibi became the standard imaging procedure worldwide for localizing hyperactive parathyroid glands.[1,17–22]

The uptake of technetium 99m Tc-sestamibi in parathyroid tissue depends on the blood flow, gland size, and the metabolic activity of the gland (in the mitochondria).[1,23] Sestamibi accumulates in the thyroid and parathyroid tissues within minutes after intravenous administration, but it has a different washout rate from these two tissues. This radiotracer is released faster from the thyroid than from the parathyroid.[1] The different washout rates in the two tissues is likely caused by a distinct expression of P-glycoprotein (an outflux system) in these two glands.[1,24–27] The dual-phase scintigraphy was originally described by Taillefer and colleagues.[19] This protocol consists of the acquisition of planar images of the neck at 15 minutes and 2 to 3 hours after the intravenous injection of sestamibi (activity 740–925 MBq). The scan is positive for a parathyroid disease if the area of increased uptake in the early images persists in the late images while the background uptake in the thyroid tissue diminishes with time.[19] This technique is relatively easy and improves the sensitivity and the specificity of the technique. It has two potential drawbacks: (1) Some solid thyroid nodules also concentrate sestamibi regardless of whether they are benign or malignant or may appear cold or hot on the thyroid scintigraphy.[1,28] This condition is particularly frequent in persons in mid-south Europe.[1] (2) On occasions, parathyroid disease can have rapid sestamibi washout similar to thyroid gland.[8]

When there is a suspicion of concomitant nodular goiter, it is useful to perform a thyroid scintigraphy along with sestamibi scan to avoid erroneous results. It can be achieved with a double tracer subtraction scintigraphy protocol. There are various double tracer subtraction scintigraphy protocols. The protocol to be used depends on (1) the kind of thyroid tracer used and (2) the sequence of administration of the two radiopharmaceuticals. The following protocols have been described for this purpose.

[123]Iodine/technetium 99m Tc-sestamibi subtraction technique

The patient is administered 10 MBq of [123]I. After 2 to 4 hours, technetium 99m Tc-sestamibi is injected and imaging is performed distinctly or at the same time using separate energy windows (140 KeV for $^{99m}TcO^{4-}$, 159 KeV for ^{123}I). The thyroid image is then subtracted from the sestamibi image.[29] This protocol is not widely used because of the high cost and limited availability of [123]I. To acquire appropriate counting statistics

for thyroid images with iodine at the doses used, a long imaging time is needed.

$^{99m}TcO^{4-}$/ technetium 99m Tc-sestamibi subtraction technique

This is a practical dual tracer subtraction technique. Patients are injected with 185 MBq of $^{99m}TcO^{4-}$, and after 20 minutes the imaging is performed. While keeping the patient in the same position, 300 MBq of sestamibi are injected, and a 20-minute dynamic acquisition is performed. The thyroid image is then subtracted from the final image. This protocol provides high sensitivity and specificity values (89% and 98%, respectively).[30] This technique does have a fault, however; the high count rate from the thyroid image, caused by the intense uptake of $^{99m}TcO^{4-}$ from the thyroid gland compared with the uptake of sestamibi, does not allow for the identification of a parathyroid adenoma located behind the thyroid contour. Geatti and colleagues[31] modified the protocol to correct this problem by reducing the dose of $^{99m}TcO^{4-}$ to 40 MBq and increasing that of sestamibi up to 400 to 500 MBq. The sensitivity rose to 95% in patients with primary hyperparathyroidism without false-positive results because of thyroid nodules.

$^{99m}TcO^{4-}$ and potassium perchlorate (KclO^{4-})/technetium 99m Tc-sestamibi

This protocol was developed in our center[32] and permits the rapid washout of $^{99m}TcO^{4-}$ from the thyroid tissue by the oral administration of KClO^{4-} 20 minutes after the intravenous injection of 150 MBq of $^{99m}TcO^{4-}$. For this protocol, before positioning the patient under the gamma-camera, 400 mg of KClO^{4-} are administered orally. Two scans are acquired—one immediately after the patient is positioned under the camera and the other after waiting for 20 minutes. After an intravenous injection of 550 MBq of sestamibi, without moving the patient from the gamma-camera, six to seven dynamic planar frames of the neck and mediastinum (generally 5 minutes per frame) are acquired. At the conclusion of the examination, one or two frames are chosen and, after proper normalization for the subtraction (sestamibi–pertechnetate), the final image is interpreted for parathyroid abnormalities. **Figs. 1** and **2** show two examples of such scans.

Technetium 99m Tc-sestamibi/$^{99m}TcO^{4-}$

In this protocol the thyroid tracer $^{99m}TcO^{4-}$ is injected at the end of a dual phase scintigraphy with sestamibi. After completion of the late (2–3 hours) sestamibi image acquisition, the patient receives $^{99m}TcO^{4-}$; after 20 minutes, the thyroid images are acquired. To obtain a "pure

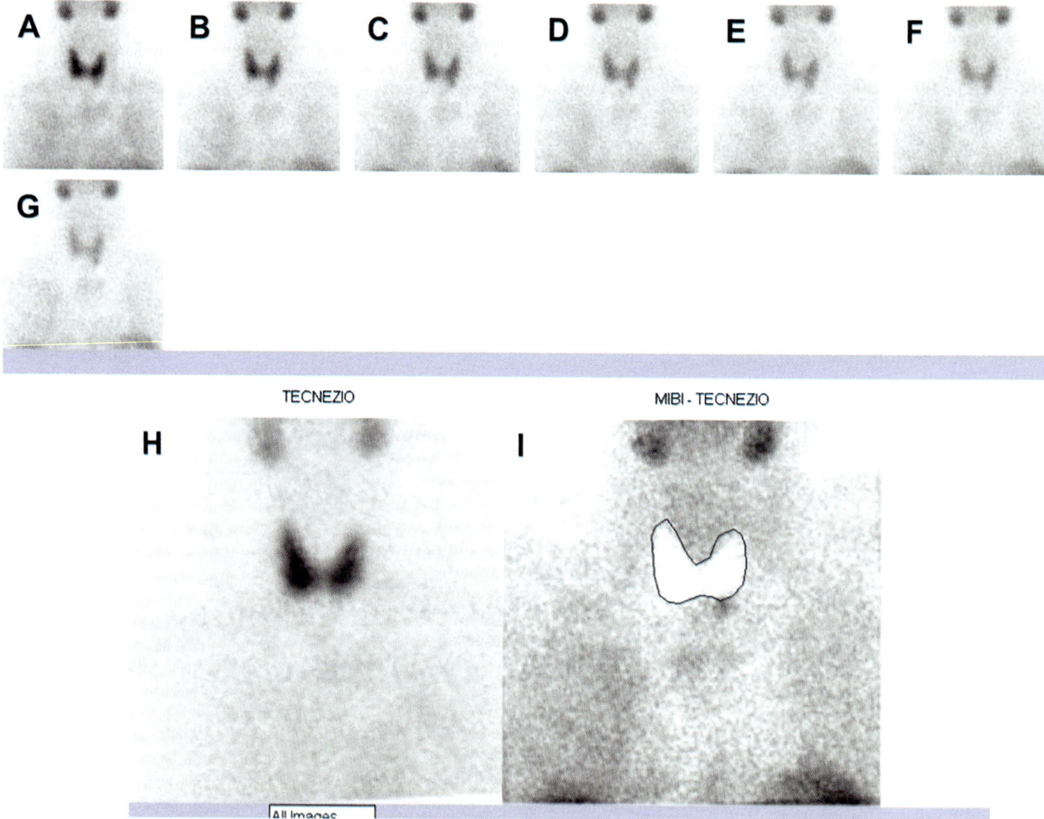

Fig. 1. Patient with primary hyperparathyroidism caused by a small (100-mg) solitary adenoma localized just behind the right thyroid lobe. (*A–G*) Dynamic sestamibi washout images, 5 minutes each. (*H*) Pertechnetate thyroid image. (*I*) Subtracted (sestamibi–pertechentate) image.

$^{99m}TcO^{4-}$" image it is necessary to subtract the late sestamibi image from the last image acquired. The pure $^{99m}TcO^{4-}$ image is used to generate the real subtraction sestamibi-$^{99m}TcO^{4-}$ scan.[1]

It is worth noting that some authors have proposed the use of technetium 99m Tc tetrofosmin as an alternative to sestamibi. These two tracers are virtually interchangeable for myocardial perfusion imaging, even if they have a different mechanism for uptake. (Sestamibi accumulates primarily in the mitochondria, and tetrofosmin is retained primarily in the citosol fraction.) This is not true for parathyroid scintigraphy; tetrofosmin can replace sestamibi only in double tracer subtraction protocols because its washout from thyroid parenchyma is considerably slower than that of sestamibi. The single tracer dual phase protocol is not always reliable with this tracer.[33–36]

We can speculate that parathyroid scintigraphy with sestamibi is the most sensitive and specific examination to localize the disease in cases of known primary hyperparathyroidism, mainly when the double tracer subtraction protocol is used.[8] The sensitivity depends on many factors: size of the gland, regional perfusion, functional activity, cell cycle phase, and prevalence of mitochondria-rich oxyphil cells.[1,37,38] To improve sensitivity, especially in patients with recurring hyperparathyroidism after prior surgery, and to better localize diseased parathyroid glands, especially when they are ectopic, some authors routinely use tomographic (SPECT) images of the neck and thorax.[1,37,39–45] SPECT is useful in minimally invasive radioguided surgery, not only for accurately localizing the gland but also for calculating the gland-to-background-uptake ratio to identify the gland during exploration with a gamma probe. This approach may allow a proper selection of patients for whom a minimally invasive approach can be offered with potential for a cure.[46–49]

The combination of parathyroid sestamibi scintigraphy with structural imaging of the neck, particularly US, has led to increased specificity. Casara and colleagues[50] used a $^{99m}TcO^{4-}$ plus $KClO^{4-}$/technetium 99m Tc-sestamibi protocol and US scan and reported a sensitivity of 94% with no false-positive results, although there was concomitant nodular goiter in 29% of the cases.

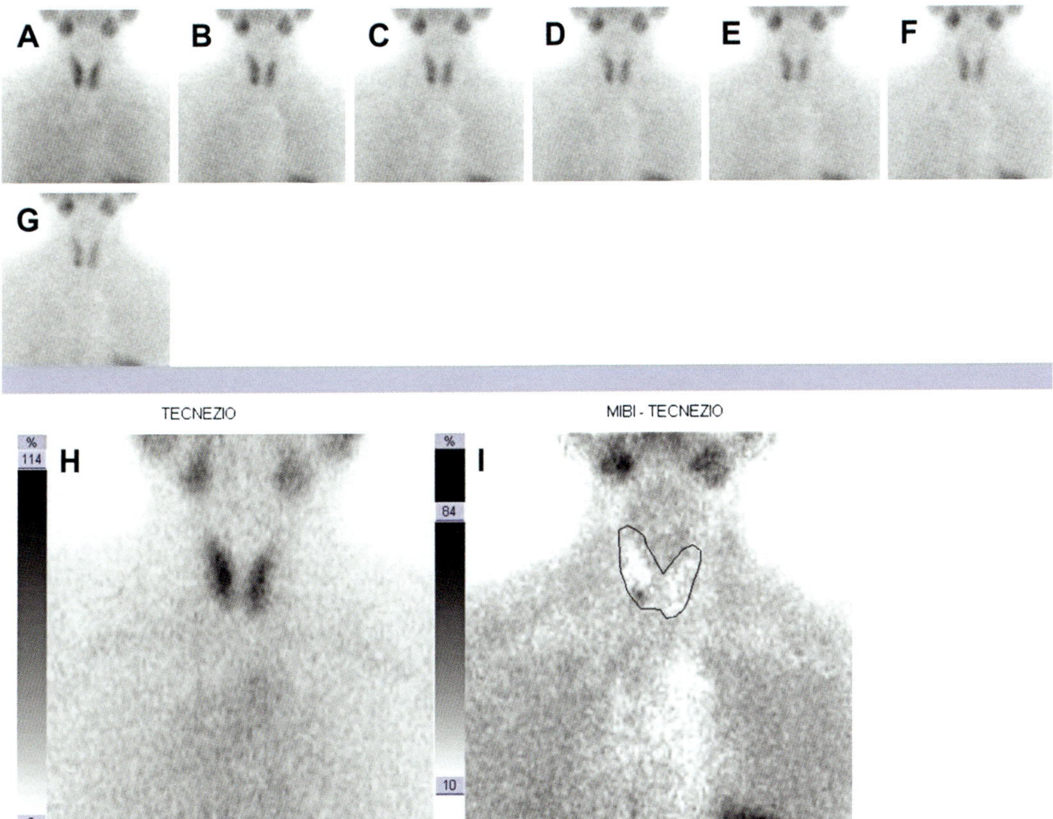

Fig. 2. Patient with primary hyperparathyroidism caused by a small 200-mg solitary adenoma localized just beyond the left thyroid lobe. (*A–G*) Dynamic sestamibi washout images, 5 minutes each. (*H*) Pertechnetate thyroid image. (*I*) Subtracted (sestamibi–pertechentate) image.

Although US has lower sensitivity and accuracy than scintigraphy for finding parathyroid tumors, in some cases US imaging serves an important function in this setting. In particular, it is used to (1) confirm the presence of a scan-positive solitary parathyroid adenoma, (2) provide additional information about the depth of the adenoma (by distinguishing parathyroid adenoma located behind and close to the thyroid gland from the sestamibi-avid thyroid nodules), (3) identify rare adenomas that are negative on parathyroid scintigraphy because of cystic transformation, and, in cases of hyperparathyroidism with multi-gland disease, (4) detect nondominant and scan-negative enlarged parathyroid glands. Finally, US allows identification of small (<1 cm) equivocal nodules for US-guided fine needle aspiration.[1] The introduction of SPECT-CT also may enhance the role of scintigraphy in assessing patients with hyperthyroidism.

Positron Emission Tomographic Imaging

2-[18F] fluoro-2-deoxy-D-glucose (FDG) is the most widely use PET radiopharmaceutical for various indications. FDG is a glucose analog that has a high sensitivity for detecting most malignant tumors and is useful for staging, re-staging, assessing therapy response, and performing follow-up.[51] Initial PET studies for detecting diseased parathyroid gland disease were performed with FDG,[5] but the results obtained were conflicting.[52,53] Some authors noted a too low sensitivity for this imaging technique and cautioned against its systematic role in preoperative detection and localization of parathyroid glands.[53] In the head-neck region, it is common to note nonspecific uptake of FDG caused by inflammatory conditions that can mimic or obscure an overactive parathyroid gland.

Lange-Nolde and colleagues[54] used [18F]-3,4-diidrossi-fenilalanina (F-DOPA) as a tracer to detect parathyroid adenomas, but they reported that none of their patients (*n* = 9) with histologically proven parathyroid adenoma showed significant uptake of [18F]-DOPA in the affected parathyroid glands. They concluded that PET with [18F]-DOPA is not useful in the detection of parathyroid adenoma in patients with primary hyperparathyroidism.[54] Currently, the only PET tracer that seems to play a role in the study of parathyroid disease is ^{11}C-methionine. ^{11}C-methionine is a neutral amino acidic that has been used successfully to study brain tumors. Unlike FDG, it does not accumulate in the healthy brain or in nonactive tissues. The most appropriate indication for its use is when conventional imaging procedures are unable to discriminate between benign conditions and recurrent cancer.[51]

Parathyroid scintigraphy with ^{11}C-methionine is not a new technique for parathyroid imaging; it was introduced approximately 40 years ago with the radioisotope ^{75}Se as the label. The success of parathyroid localization was variable with this tracer and was subsequently supplanted by other radiopharmaceuticals, as noted previously.[8] The reintroduction of ^{11}C-labeled methionine as a parathyroid

PET agent has resulted in interest in this compound for examining primary, secondary, tertiary, and recurrent primary hyperparathyroidism.[16]

Accumulation of ^{11}C-methionine in the parathyroid tissue is affected by the size of the lesion, amino acid influx (transmembrane transport), protein synthesis, and methionine donor transmethylation of the abnormally stimulated parathyroid gland.[5,16,55] In particular, at the pathophysiologic level, the high uptake of ^{11}C-methionine by the hyperfunctioning parathyroid tissue may be explained by some characteristics in the intermediary metabolism, namely that of the synthesis of the precursor hormone pre-pro-PTH, which needs seven methionine residues for its synthesis.[6]

Based on what is published in the literature, no comparison has been made between conventional

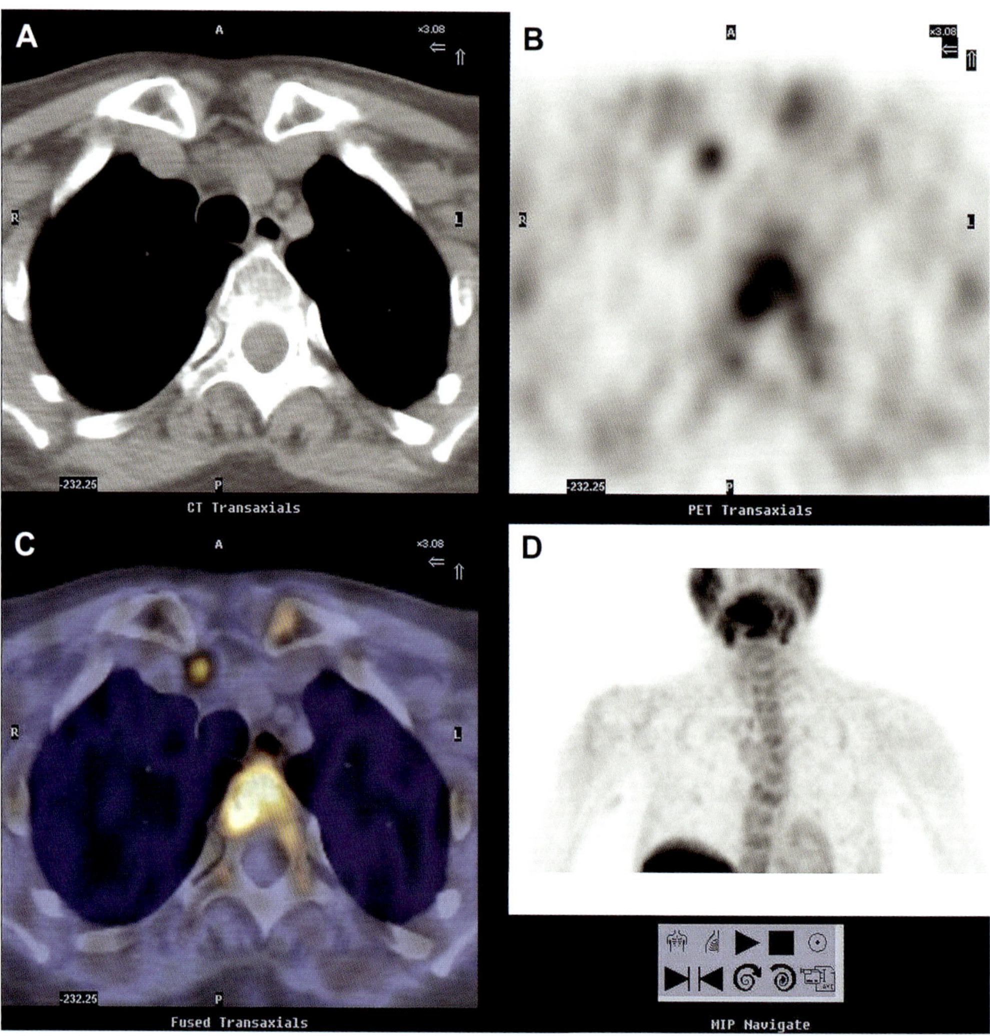

Fig. 3. Primary hyperparathyroid patient with a small (140-mg) parathyroid gland located behind the right thyroid lobe clearly depicted at ^{11}C-methionine PET/CT. Sestamibi scan and ultrasound produced negative results in this case. (*A*) CT scan. (*B*) PET scan. (*C*) Fusion image. (*D*) MIP image.

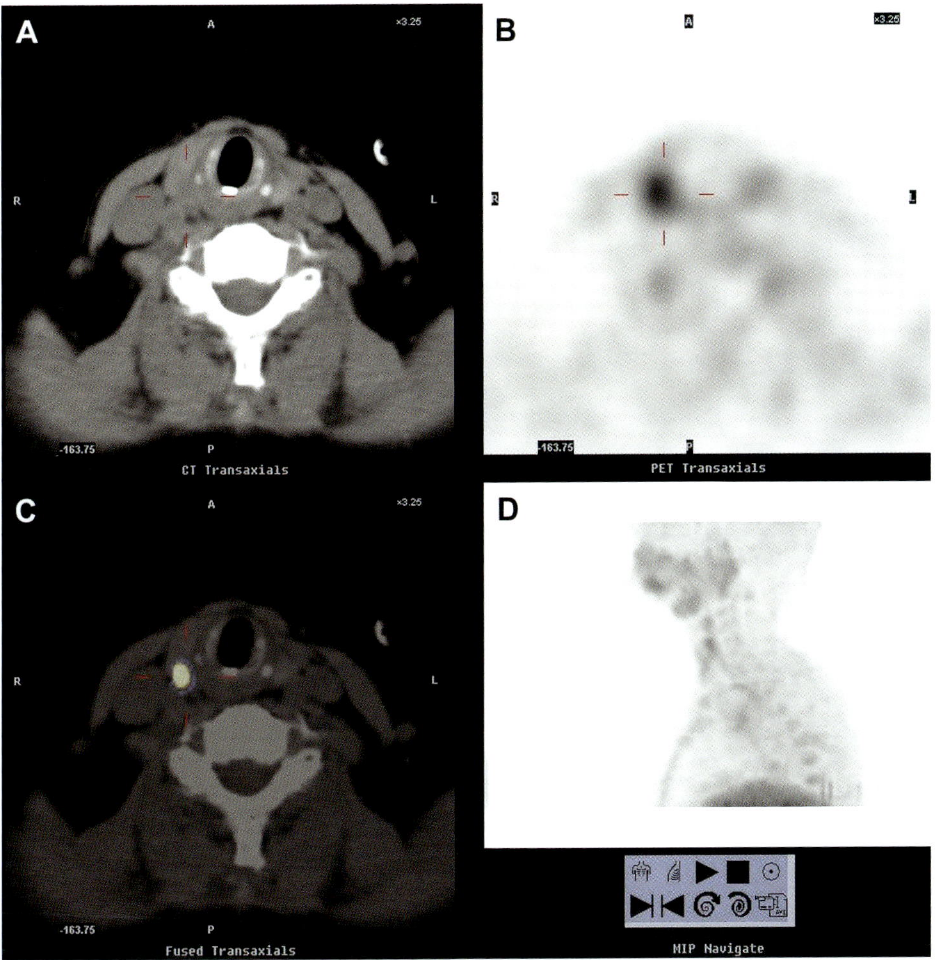

Fig. 4. Recurrent primary hyperparathyroid patient with a small (90 mg) parathyroid gland located beyond the right thyroid lobe clearly depicted at ^{11}C-methionine PET/CT. Sestamibi scan and ultrasound were negative in this case. (*A*) CT scan; (*B*) PET scan; (*C*) fusion image; (*D*) MIP image.

scintigraphy and ^{11}C-methionine–based PET imaging for imaging parathyroid lesions. ^{11}C-methionine PET seems to be an optimal imaging technique for this purpose. Some authors reported that it provides more accurate results than sestamibi, particularly in cases of primary hyperparathyroidism (adenoma).[5] ^{11}C-methionine PET also yields positive results in cases of recurrent primary hyperparathyroidism and in the presence of secondary hyperparathyroidism, where classical sestamibi scintigraphy has failed.[6,16] ^{11}C-methionine PET, compared with sestamibi, has the advantage of better spatial and contrast resolution. It is estimated that the lower limit of detection of parathyroid adenoma by ^{11}C-methionine is approximately 200 mg[16,55] versus 500 mg with sestamibi.[16] This finding is not surprising because PET is substantially superior to planar and tomographic imaging with single emitting radiopharmaceuticals.

The introduction of PET-CT imaging to this day-to-day practice of medicine further enhances the role of this technique in complicated settings, such as those encountered in patients who have hyperparathyroidism.

Unfortunately, ^{11}C has a short half-life (approximately 20 minutes), and the production of ^{11}C-methionine needs close proximity to a cyclotron and the ability for a fast synthesis technique. This tracer is only available in a few centers at this time. **Figs. 3** and **4** show two examples of ^{11}C-methionine PET/CT in hyperparathyroidism with negative results on sestamibi scans.

SUMMARY

In parathyroid disease, classical scintigraphic techniques remain the first choice for localizing hyperfunctional parathyroid glands in primary known hyperparathyroidism and in case of secondary, tertiary, and recurrent hyperparathyroidism. When classical scintigraphic techniques are not diagnostic, however, ^{11}C-methionine seems to offer a good imaging alternative.

REFERENCES

1. Mariani G, Gulec SA, Rubello D, et al. Preoperative localization and radioguided parathyroid surgery. J Nucl Med 2003;44:1443–58.
2. Elgazzar A. The pathophysiologic basis of nuclear medicine. Heidelberg, Germany: Springer; 2001. ch.7. p. 141–6.
3. Doppman J. Reoperative parathyroid surgery: localization procedures, parathyroid surgery. Prog Surg 1986;18:117–36.
4. O'Doherty MJ, Kettle AG. Parathyroid imaging: preoperative localisation. Nucl Med Commun 2003; 24:125–31.
5. Beggs AD, Hain SF. Localization of parathyroid adenomas using 11C-methionine positron emission tomography. Nucl Med Commun 2005;26:133–6.
6. Otto D, Boerne AR, Hofmann M, et al. Pre-operative localization of hyperfunctional parathyroid tissue with 11C-methionine PET. Eur J Nucl Med Mol Imaging 2004;31:1405–12.
7. Giordano A, Rubello D, Casara D. New trends in parathyroid scintigraphy. Eur J Nucl Med 2001;28: 1409–20.
8. Rubello D. How should the "optimal" pre-operative localizing imaging work-up in hyperparathyroid patients be? J Endocrinol Invest 2006;29(9):854–6.
9. Erdman WA, Breslan NA, Weinreb JC, et al. Noninvasive localization of parathyroid adenomas: a comparison of X-ray computerized tomography, ultrasound, scintigraphy and MRI. Magn Reson Imaging 1989m;7:187–94.
10. Auffermann W, Gooding GAW, Okerlund MD, et al. Diagnosis of recurrent hyperparathyroidism: comparison of MR imaging and other imaging techniques. Am J Roentgenol 1988;150:1027–33.
11. Peck WW, Higgins CR, Fisher MR, et al. Hypeparathyroidism: comparison of MR imaging with radionuclide scanning. Radiology 1987;163:415–20.
12. Levin KE, Gooding GAW, Okerland M, et al. Localizing studies in patients with persistent or recurrent hyperparathyroidism. Surgery 1987;102:917–25.
13. Miller DL, Doppman JR, Shawker TH, et al. Localization of parathyroid adenomas in patients who have undergone surgery. Part 1. Noninvasive imaging methods. Radiology 1987;162:133–7.
14. Coakley AJ. Nuclear medicine and parathyroid surgery: a change in practice. Nucl Med Commun 2003;24:111–3.
15. Kumar A, Cozens NJA, Nash JR. Sestamibi scan-directed unilateral neck exploration for primary hyperparathyroidism due to a solitary adenoma. Eur J Surg Oncol 2000;26:785–8.
16. Rubello D, Fanti S, Nanni C, et al. 11C-methionine PET/CT in 99mTc-sestamibi-negative hyperparathyroidism in patient with renal failure on chronic haemodialysis. Eur J Nucl Med Mol Imaging 2006; 33:453–9.
17. Coakley AJ, Kettle AG, Wells CP, et al. 99mTcmsestamibi: a new agent for parathyroid imaging. Nucl Med Commun 1989;10:791–4.
18. O'Doherty MJ, Kettle AG, Wells P, et al. Parathyroid imaging with technetium-99m-sestamibi: preoperative localization and tissue uptake studies. J Nucl Med 1992;33:313–9.
19. Taillefer R, Boucher Y, Potvin C, et al. Detection and localization of parathyroid adenomas in patients with hyperparathyroidism using a single radionuclide imaging procedure with technetium-99m-sestamibi (double phase study). J Nucl Med 1992;33(10): 1801–7.
20. Webwer CJ, Vansant J, Alazraki N, et al. Value of technetium-99m-sestamibi iodine imaging in reoperative parathyroid surgery. Surgery 1993;114: 1011–8.
21. Casas AT, Burke GJ, Mansberg AR, et al. Impact of technetium-99m-sestamibi localization on operative time and success of operation for primary hyperparathyroidism. Am Surg 1994;60:12–7.
22. Feingold DL, Alexander HR, Chen CC, et al. Ultrasound and sestamibi scan as the only preoperative imaging test in reoperation for parathyroid adenomas. Surgery 2000;128:1103–10.
23. Hetrakul N, Civelek AC, Stag CA, et al. In vitro accumulation of technetium-99m-sestamibi in human parathyroid mitochondria. Surgery 2001;130: 1011–8.
24. Piwnica-Worms D, Chiu ML, Budding M, et al. Functional imaging of multidrug resistant P-glycoprotein with organotechnetium complex. Cancer Res 1993; 53:977–84.
25. Mitchell BK, Cornelius EA, Zoghbi S, et al. Mechanism of technetium 99m sestamibi parathyroid imaging and possible role of p-glycoprotein. Surgery 1996;120:1039–45.
26. Bhatnagar A, Vezza PR, Bryan JA, et al. Technetium-99m-sestamibi parathyroid scintigraphy: effect of P-glycoprotein, histology and tumor size on detectability. J Nucl Med 1998;39:1617–20.
27. Yamaguchi S, Yachiku S, Hashimoto H, et al. Relation between technetium 99m methoxyisobutylisonitrile accumulation and multidrug resistance protein in the parathyroid glands. World J Surg 2002;26:29–34.
28. Foldes I, Levay A, Stotz G. Comparative scanning of thyroid nodules with technetium-99m pertechnetate and technetiun-99m-nethoxyisobutylisonitrile. Eur J Nucl Med 1993;20:330–3.

29. Hindie E, Melliere D, Jeanguillame C, et al. Parathyroid imaging using simultaneous double window recording of technetium-99m-sestamibi and iodine-123. J Nucl Med 1998;39:1100–5.

30. Casara D, Rubello D, Saladini G, et al. Imaging procedures in evaluation of hyperparathyroidism: the role of scintigraphy with 99mTc-MIBI. In: Rvelli E, Samori G, editors. Primary and secondary hyperparathyroidism. Milan (Italy): Wichtig Editore; 1992. p. 133–6.

31. Geatti O, Shapiro B, Orsolon P, et al. Localization of parathyroid enlargement: experience with technetium 99m methoxyisobutylisonitrile and thallium-201 scintigraphy, ultrasound and computed tomography. Eur J Nucl Med 1994;21:17–23.

32. Rubello D, Saladini G, Casara D, et al. Parathyroid imaging with pertechnetate plus perchlorate/MIBI subtraction scintigraphy: a fast and effective technique. Clin Nucl Med 2000;25:527–31.

33. Fjield JG, Erichsen K, Pfeffer PF, et al. Technetium-99m-tetrofosmin for parathyroid scintigraphy: a comparison with sestamibi. J Nucl Med 1997;38:831–4.

34. O'Doherty MJ. Radionuclide parathyroid imaging. J Nucl Med 1997;38:840–1.

35. Gallowitsch HJ, Mikosch P, Kresnik E, et al. Comparison between 99mTc-tetrofosmin/pertechnetate subtraction scintigraphy and 99mTc-tetrofosmin SPECT for preoperative localization of parathyroid adenoma in an endemic goiter area. Invest Radiol 2000;35:453–9.

36. Froeberg AC, Valkema R, Bonjer HJ, et al. 99mTc-tetrofosmin or 99mTc-sestamibi for double-phase parathyroid scintigraphy? Eur J Nucl Med 2003;30:193–6.

37. Torregrosa JV, Fernandez-Cruz L, Canaleyo A, et al. 99mTc-sestamibi scintigraphy and cell cycle in parathyroid glands of secondary hyperparathyroidism. World J Surg 2000;24:1386–90.

38. Carpentier A, Jeannotte S, Verreault J, et al. Preoperative localization of parathyroid lesions in hyperparathyroidism: relationship between technetium-99n-MIBI uptake and oxyphil cell content. J Nucl Med 1998;39:1441–4.

39. Uden P, Aspelin P, Berglund J. Preoperative localization in unilateral parathyroid surgery: a cost-benefit study on ultrasound, computed tomography and scintigraphy. Acta Chir Scand 1990;156:29–35.

40. Lloyd MN, Lees WR, Milroy EJ. Preoperative localisation in primary hyperparathyroidism. Clin Radiol 1990;41:239–43.

41. Billotey C, Sarfati E, Aurengo A, et al. Advantages of SPECT in technetium-99m-sestamibi parathyroid scintigraphy. J Nucl Med 1996;37:1773–8.

42. Francis IS, Loney EL, Buscombe JR, et al. Technetium-99n-sestamibi dual phase SPECT imaging: concordance with ultrasound. Nucl Med Commun 1999;20:487–8.

43. Pattou F, Huglo D, Proye C. Radionuclide scanning in parathyroid disease. Br J Surg 1998m;85:1605–16.

44. Loney EL, Buscombe JR, Hilson AJW, et al. Preoperative imaging of parathyroid glands. Lancet 1999;354:1819–20.

45. Moka D, Voth E, Dietlein M, et al. Technetium 99m-NIBI-SPECT: a highly sensitive diagnostic tool for localization of parathyroid adenomas. Surgery 2000;128:29–35.

46. Rubello D, Massaro A, Cittadin S, et al. Role of 99mTc-sestamibi SPECT in accurate selection of primary hyperparathyroid patients for minimally invasive radio-guided surgery. Eur J Nucl Med Mol Imaging 2006;33:1091–4.

47. Rubello D, Pelizzo MR, Boni G, et al. Radioguided surgery of primary hyperparathyroidism using the low-dose 99mTc-sestamibi protocol: multi-institutional experience from the Italian Study Group on Radioguided Surgery and Immunoscintigraphy (GISCRIS). J Nucl Med 2005;46(2):220–6.

48. Rubello D, Piotto A, Casara D, et al. Role of gamma probes in performing minimally invasive parathyroidectomy in patients with primary hyperparathyroidism: optimization of preoperative and intraoperative procedures. Eur J Endocrinol 2003;149(1):7–15.

49. Rubello D, Pelizzo MR, Casara D. Nuclear medicine and minimally invasive surgery of parathyroid adenomas: a fair marriage. Eur J Nucl Med Mol Imaging 2003;30(2):189–92.

50. Casara D, Rubello D, Pelizzo NR, et al. Clinical role of 99mTcOS/MIBI scan, ultrasound and intra-operative gamma probe in the performance of unilateral and minimally invasive surgery in primary hyperparathyroidism. Eur J Nucl Med 2001;28:1351–9.

51. Nanni C, Rubello D, Al-Nahhas A, et al. Clinical PET in oncology: not only FDG. Nucl Med Commun 2006;27:685–8.

52. Neumann DR, Esselstyn CB, MacIntyre WJ, et al. Comparison of FDG-PET and sestamibi SPECT in primary hyperparathyroidism. J Nucl Med 1996;37:1809–15.

53. Melon P, Luxen A, Hamoir E, et al. Fluorine 18-fluorodeoxyglucose positron emission tomography for preoperative parathyroid imaging in primary hyperparathyroidism. Eur J Nucl Med 1995;22:556–8.

54. Lange-Nolde A, Zajic T, Slawik M, et al. PET with 18F-DOPA in the imaging of parathyroid adenoma in patients with primary hyperparathyroidism: a pilot study. Nucklearmedizin 2006;45:193–6.

55. Sundin A, Johansson C, Hellman P, et al. PET and parathyroid L-[Carbon-11] methionine accumulation in hyperparathyroidism. J Nucl Med 1996;37:1766–70.

The Role of CT, MR Imaging, and Ultrasonography in Endocrinology

Drew A. Torigian, MD, MA*, Geming Li, MD, Abass Alavi, MD, PhD

KEYWORDS
- Computed tomography (CT)
- Magnetic resonance (MR) imaging
- Ultrasonography (US)
- Endocrinology • Endocrine • Pituitary
- Thyroid • Parathyroid • Adrenal

CT, MR imaging, and ultrasonography are tomographic structural imaging modalities commonly used to evaluate the organs of the endocrine system. CT makes use of x-rays, MR imaging uses radiofrequency waves and magnetism, and ultrasonography employs sound waves. The signals obtained from the various tissues or lesions of the body through these imaging modalities are described in terms of attenuation in the case of CTs, signal intensity (SI) in the case of MR images, and echogenicity in the case of ultrasonography. These signals are useful for grossly characterizing tissue composition, and can be enhanced through intravenously administered contrast agents (iodine-based for CT, gadolinium-based for MR images, and microbubble-based for ultrasonography).[1]

These imaging modalities have the advantages of high spatial resolution, multiplanar tomographic or volumetric image display, and relatively short examination times (typically on the order of 5–10 minutes for CT, 20–30 minutes for MR imaging, and 10–20 minutes for ultrasonography). CT and MR images have the additional advantages of whole body coverage (related to multidetector row and parallel imaging technologies, respectively), good soft tissue contrast between normal structures and disease processes (such contrast is greater with MR images than with CT), and

operator independence.[2,3] CT can be used when there are contraindications to MR imaging, such as presence of a transvenous pacemaker, intracranial ferromagnetic aneurysm clips, or orbital metallic foreign bodies.[4] Similarly, MR imaging can be used when there are contraindications to administration of iodinated contrast material (such as an allergy to iodinated contrast), and allows for the acquisition of multiple image sequences (T1-weighted [T1-W] and T2-weighted [T2-W]) that may be useful to depict different characteristics of disease processes affecting the endocrine organs. MR imaging is therefore frequently used as a problem-solving tool to better delineate the nature and extent of disease.

Unfortunately, CT has the disadvantage in its use of ionizing radiation, which has implications for the imaging evaluation of patients, especially children, young adults, and pregnant women.[5] Moreover, intravenous contrast agent administration for use with CT and MR imaging is contraindicated in the setting of pregnancy and in the presence of renal insufficiency or failure. The latter is associated with the risk of exacerbation of renal dysfunction following administration of iodinated contrast material and risk of induction of nephrogenic systemic fibrosis, a serious and potentially fatal medical condition, following administration of gadolinium-based contrast material.[6,7]

Department of Radiology, Hospital of the University of Pennsylvania, 3400 Spruce Street, Philadelphia, PA 19104-4283, USA
* Corresponding author.
E-mail address: drew.torigian@uphs.upenn.edu (D. Torigian).

PET Clin 2 (2008) 395–408
doi:10.1016/j.cpet.2008.05.002

Ultrasonography has the additional advantages of low cost, color Doppler imaging capability (for gross assessment of tissue perfusion), real-time image acquisition, portability, and absence of ionizing radiation (similar to MR imaging). However, ultrasonography has the disadvantages of inferior soft tissue contrast compared with CT and MR imaging, limited depth of penetration due to attenuation of sound waves by intervening tissue (particularly in obese patients), occasional inability to find an acoustic window between sound wave attenuating structures (bone, lung, and air-filled bowel) to perform ultrasonographic imaging, frequent nonspecificity of detected abnormalities for definitive characterization of a disease process, and operator dependence with regard to image acquisition, image quality, and disease detection.[8]

Dual-energy CT; diffusion-weighted MR imaging; dynamic enhanced CT, MR imaging, and ultrasound perfusion imaging; magnetic resonance spectroscopy; tissue harmonic imaging; and other advanced functionalities of CT, MR imaging, and ultrasonography with regard to gross functional imaging of the endocrine organs of the body are feasible as well in clinical practice and may add value in the diagnostic study of patients with endocrine disorders. However, these are beyond the scope of this article.

STRUCTURAL IMAGING OF THE PITUITARY GLAND

Unenhanced head CT is generally the first-line structural imaging test for evaluating patients who present with symptoms or signs thought to be related to disease of the intracranial contents, although detected abnormalities within the region of the sella turcica are usually nonspecific in appearance. In patients with pituitary macroadenoma and other large sellar lesions, CT is also superior to MR imaging for assessment of the adjacent osseous structures, such as the sellar floor.[9] However, in general, if the patient has a known abnormality involving the pituitary gland, hypothalamus, or sella turcica, or has neurologic or hormonal symptoms or signs suggestive of disease involving these structures, then MR imaging will typically be used as the first-line structural imaging test because it has high spatial resolution, high contrast resolution, and multiplanar image acquisition capability. These strengths allow for improved distinction between pituitary lesions and extrapituitary sellar and suprasellar lesions, as well as improved delineation of the size and shape of pituitary lesions, the presence of cavernous sinus extension, the presence of hemorrhagic or cystic change, and of the positional relationship

with the optic pathways.[10] MR imaging is also useful after therapeutic intervention to assess for postsurgical complications as well as for the presence of residual or recurrent disease, and specialized MR imaging techniques may additionally improve the management of patients with pituitary lesions.[11,12] Ultrasonography is generally not used to evaluate the pituitary gland or sellar region in adults because no acoustic window in the calvarium exists through which to perform imaging.

Pituitary adenomas, the most common cause of masses in the sella turcica in adults, are tumors of the anterior pituitary gland and are almost always benign. They account for up to 10% of intracranial neoplasms.[13,14] Those lesions less than 1 cm in diameter are called microadenomas, whereas those that are 1 cm or more in diameter are called macroadenomas.[14] On CT, pituitary adenomas are typically hypoattenuating compared with the normal pituitary gland on both unenhanced and contrast-enhanced images, and may be associated with sellar floor erosion or destruction as well as focal convexity of the superior aspect of the pituitary gland (**Fig. 1**).[10] On MR imaging, pituitary adenomas appear as focal mass lesions in the pituitary gland, typically with low T1-W SI, and may contain nonenhancing areas of very high T2-W SI cystic change or areas of high T1-W and low T2-W SI hemorrhage. There may also be associated pituitary gland asymmetry, pituitary stalk deviation, or enlargement of the sella turcica with or without involvement of adjacent structures, such as the cavernous sinus and optic chiasm (see **Fig. 1**).[10,15] Furthermore, these lesions appear hypovascular relative to adjacent areas of normal pituitary tissue on contrast-enhanced T1-W images (**Fig. 2**).[16,17]

Other pituitary conditions, including hyperplasia (particularly during pregnancy), lymphocytic infiltration (usually during late pregnancy or in the postpartum period), abscess (which is rare), infarction (usually after substantial blood loss during childbirth), and other malignancies, such as primary carcinoma (which is rare), germ cell tumor (usually in children and young adults frequently associated with elevated serum beta human chorionic gonadotropin or alpha fetoprotein), lymphoma, or metastatic tumor (most commonly from breast cancer in women and lung cancer in men), may also less commonly involve the pituitary gland, although their imaging appearances on CT and MR imaging are often nonspecific.[14,18–24]

In general, whenever a sellar mass or an incidental pituitary lesion of 1 cm or more in diameter is encountered, laboratory testing of hypothalamic-pituitary hormonal function is performed, as

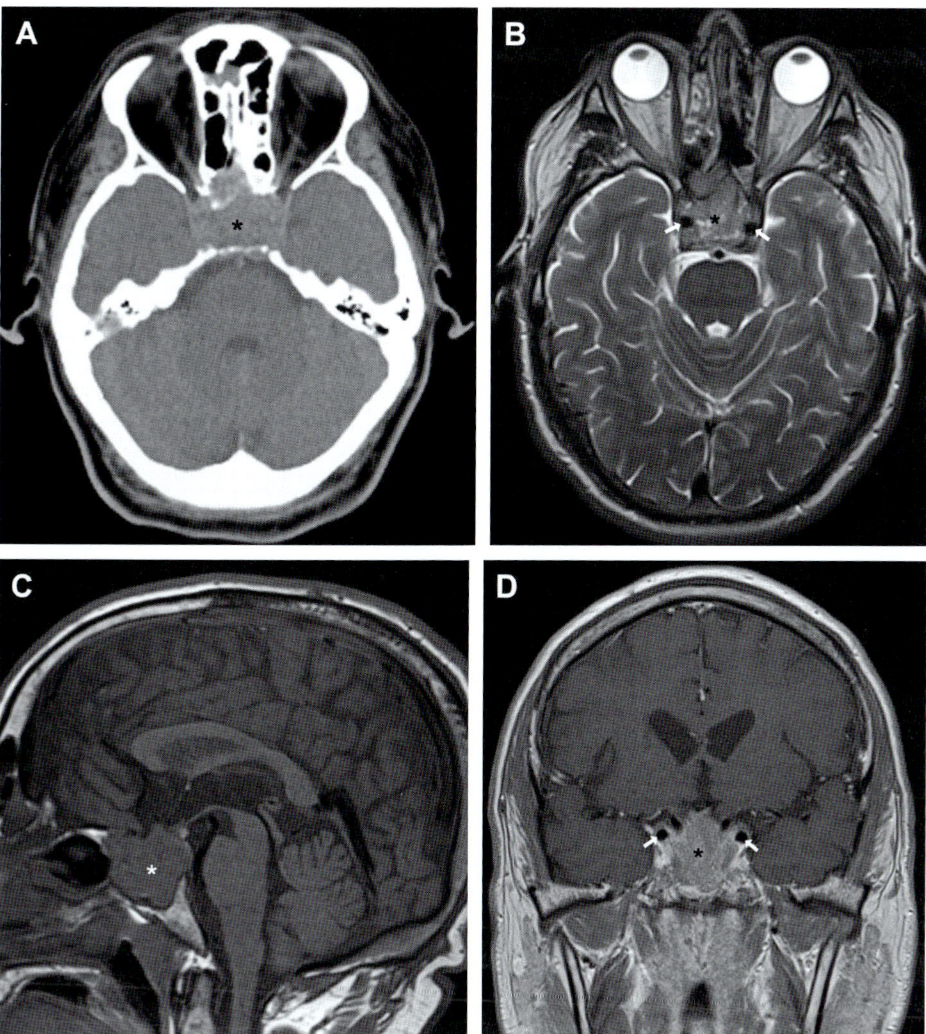

Fig. 1. Fifty-three-year-old man with history of chronic headaches and hypertension due to pituitary macroadenoma. (*A*) Axial unenhanced head CT image demonstrates large soft tissue mass (*asterisk*) centered in sella turcica with anterior extension into sphenoidal and posterior ethmoidal sinuses and lateral extension to cavernous sinuses bilaterally. Axial T2-W (*B*), sagittal T1-W (*C*), and coronal contrast-enhanced T1-W (*D*) MR images through mass (*asterisks*) reveal partial encasement of cavernous portions of internal carotid arteries (*arrows*), anterior extension to sphenoidal sinus, superior extension to suprasellar space, and scalloping and widening of sella turcica.

hormonal hypersecretion is highly suggestive of a pituitary adenoma. When an incidental pituitary lesion less than 1 cm in diameter is detected in an asymptomatic patient (in up to 10% of healthy individuals), measurement of serum prolactin levels only is recommended.[25,26] Hormonal hyposecretion may be due to any hypothalamic or pituitary lesion, and is therefore not characteristic for any particular abnormality involving these structures, although spontaneous development of central diabetes insipidus is suggestive of a lesion involving the hypothalamus or hypothalamic stalk.

STRUCTURAL IMAGING OF THE THYROID AND PARATHYROID GLANDS

Ultrasonography is the major structural imaging tool used to evaluate for disorders of the thyroid and parathyroid glands, and to provide imaging guidance for percutaneous tissue sampling of lesions involving these organs. CT and MR imaging can demonstrate the presence of focal and diffuse thyroid or parathyroid abnormalities, but the imaging findings are frequently nonspecific for definitive characterization of the underlying pathologies.

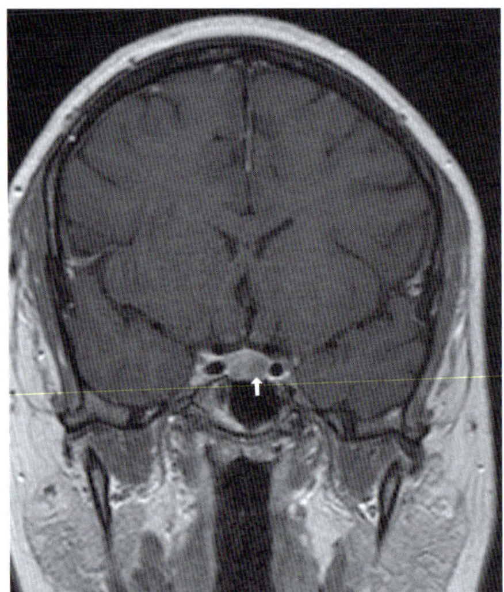

Fig. 2. Twenty-eight-year-old woman with history of hyperprolactinemia due to pituitary microadenoma. Coronal contrast-enhanced T1-W MR image through pituitary gland shows subtle 6-mm hypovascular lesion (*arrow*) in left side of pituitary gland.

These structural imaging modalities are complementary with thyroid scintigraphy and thyroid function testing.

Indications for structural imaging of the thyroid gland include a suspected thyroid nodule based on abnormal findings from prior physical examination or other imaging tests, or screening in patients with an increased risk for development of thyroid malignancies. Thyroid nodules are very common. They are found in 4% to 8% of adults on physical examination, in 10% to 41% at ultrasound, and in 50% at pathologic examination at autopsy. They also increase in prevalence with age, and are most commonly benign.[27–30] Malignancy is more common in nodules in patients younger than 20 or older than 60 years of age, in patients with a history of neck irradiation or a family history of thyroid cancer, and with physical examination findings of nodule firmness, rapid growth, fixation to adjacent structures, vocal cord paralysis, and regional lymphadenopathy. Overall, the incidence of thyroid cancer in patients with thyroid nodules selected for fine needle aspiration is 9.2% to 13.0%, no matter how many nodules are present, and, in about one third of patients with multiple thyroid nodules, the cancer is in a nondominant nodule.[31] The majority (75%–80%) of thyroid cancers are papillary type cancers. Other histologic types include follicular (10%–20%), medullary (3%–5%), and anaplastic (1%–2%).[32,33]

On ultrasound, nodule size is not predictive of malignancy, but presence of calcifications, hypoechogenicity, irregular margins, absence of a surrounding hypoechoic halo, predominantly solid composition, intranodule vascularity, and rapid growth are associated with an increased risk of thyroid cancer. However, the sensitivities, specificities, and positive and negative predictive values for these criteria are extremely variable from study to study, and no ultrasound feature has both a high sensitivity and a high positive predictive value for thyroid cancer (**Fig. 3**). Furthermore, color Doppler ultrasound cannot be used to diagnose or exclude malignancy with a high

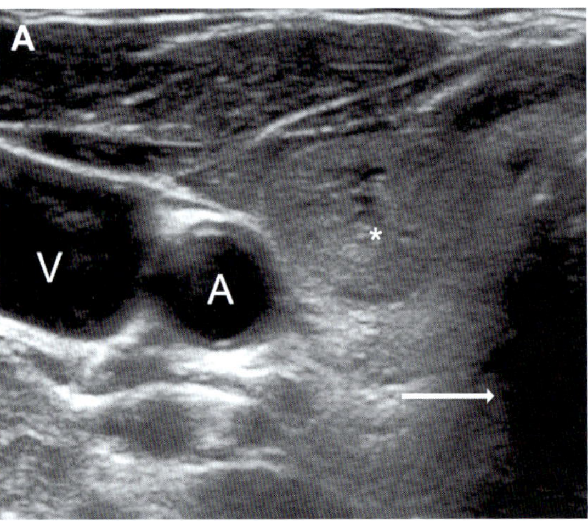
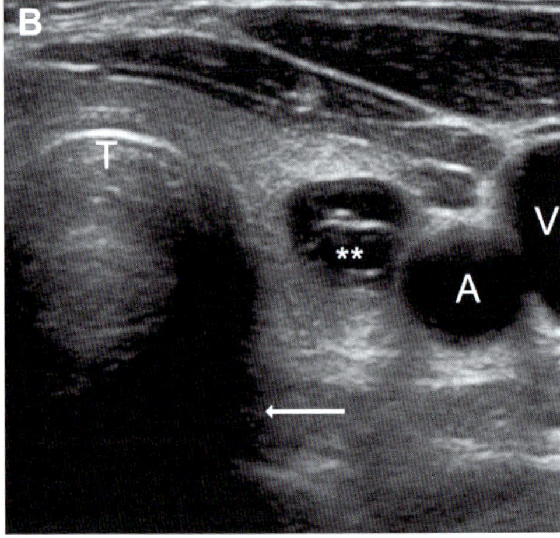

Fig. 3. Fifty-six-year-old man with history of thyroid nodules due to benign hyperplastic and adenomatous nodules. (*A* and *B*) Axial gray-scale ultrasound images through thyroid gland demonstrate hypoechoic solid thyroid nodule (*single asterisk*) in right lobe and predominantly anechoic cystic and solid thyroid nodule (*double asterisk*) in left lobe. Note anechoic internal carotid arteries (A) and internal jugular veins (V) as well as posterior acoustic shadowing (*arrows*) due to poor transmission of sound waves through air-filled trachea (T).

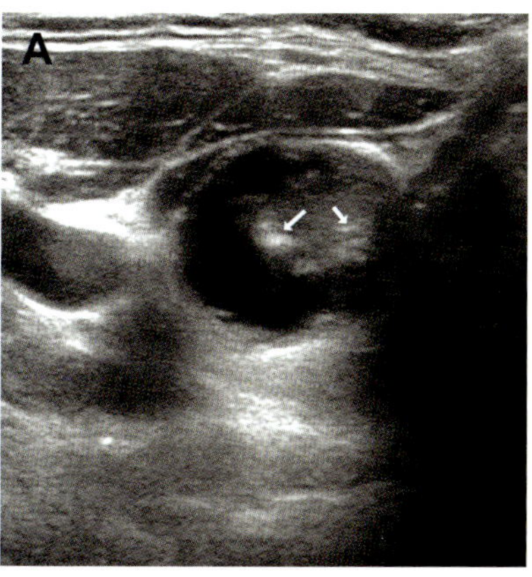
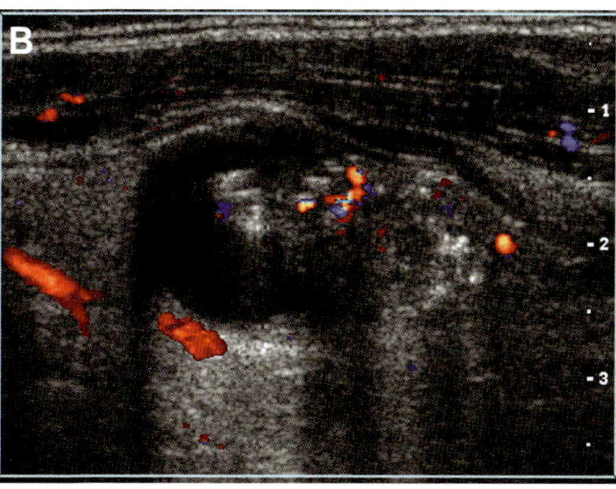

Fig. 4. Sixty-year-old man with history of solitary thyroid nodule due to papillary thyroid carcinoma. (*A*) Axial gray-scale ultrasound image through right lobe of thyroid gland reveals dominant nodule with anechoic cystic and hypoechoic solid components. Echogenic foci (*arrows*) within solid component represent microcalcifications. (*B*) Axial color Doppler ultrasound image through nodule shows intranodular vascularity.

degree of confidence, although detection of predominantly internal or central blood flow increases the chance for the presence of malignancy (**Fig. 4**).[31,34] Fine needle aspiration and cytopathologic evaluation comprise the accepted method for screening of a thyroid nodule for cancer, are safe and inexpensive, and have a high accuracy rate in the hands of an experienced cytologist, particularly when used in conjunction with ultrasound guidance to increase diagnostic yield. Furthermore, they have led to the improved detection of thyroid cancer, to decreased frequency of thyroid surgery, and to increased cancer rates at thyroidectomy.[35–38]

Ultrasonography is also the main structural imaging modality used to evaluate patients with suspected parathyroid abnormalities related to hyperparathyroidism or a palpable neck mass, and for preoperative localization of a known parathyroid adenoma to simplify and decrease the time of surgery. If one parathyroid gland is enlarged, then parathyroid adenoma (and rarely carcinoma) is the main diagnostic consideration, whereas if all four parathyroid glands are enlarged, then parathyroid hyperplasia is most likely. In general, the sensitivity of ultrasonography for parathyroid adenoma is 70% to 90%, and false-positive results may occur because of cervical lymph nodes,

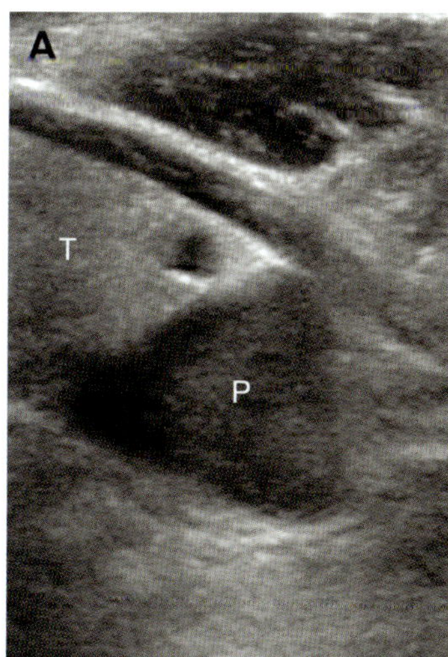
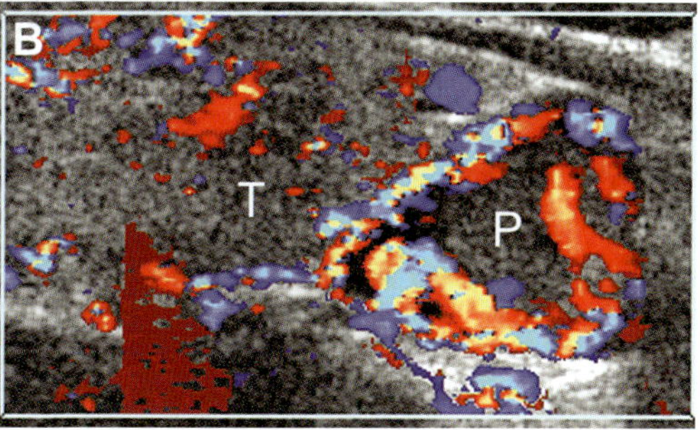

Fig. 5. Fifty-four-year-old woman with history of primary hyperparathyroidism due to parathyroid adenoma. (*A*) Sagittal gray-scale ultrasound image through thyroid gland demonstrates large hypoechoic parathyroid lesion (P) posterior and inferior to lower pole of thyroid gland (T). (*B*) Sagittal color Doppler ultrasound image through parathyroid lesion (P) shows marked hypervascularity. (T) Thyroid gland.

thyroid nodules, or misinterpretation of normal anatomic structures, such as the esophagus or longus colli muscle.[39]

On ultrasonography, a parathyroid adenoma typically appears as a homogeneously hypoechoic oval or bean-shaped lesion relative to the adjacent thyroid parenchyma with its long axis oriented in the craniocaudal direction. Color Doppler ultrasound imaging often reveals hypervascularity in the lesion as well (**Fig. 5**). Ultrasonography may also be useful to identify foci of parathyroid tissue that are present ectopically in the retrotracheal region, tracheoesophageal groove, and carotid sheath, whereas CT and MR imaging are useful to identify enhancing foci of ectopic parathyroid tissue in the mediastinum or other locations in the neck or chest, particularly when used in conjunction with parathyroid scintigraphy, single photon emission CT, or positron emission tomography.[39–41]

CT and MR imaging are more frequently used to evaluate the extent of local and distant disease in the setting of known thyroid or parathyroid malignancy, are particularly useful following surgical or radiation therapy when there is distortion of normal anatomy, and are complementary with molecular imaging techniques, such as planar nuclear scintigraphy, single photon emission CT, or positron emission tomography.[1] In particular, CT is very useful to evaluate the lungs for involvement by metastatic disease from thyroid or parathyroid carcinoma and to evaluate the trachea and bronchi for luminal compromise by extrinsic or endoluminal lesions, whereas MR imaging is useful to evaluate the muscles and bone marrow for involvement by metastatic disease (**Fig. 6**).[40,41] Intravenous iodinated contrast material administered during CT interferes with future thyroid uptake of diagnostic and therapeutic iodine radioisotopes for 2 months, and therefore

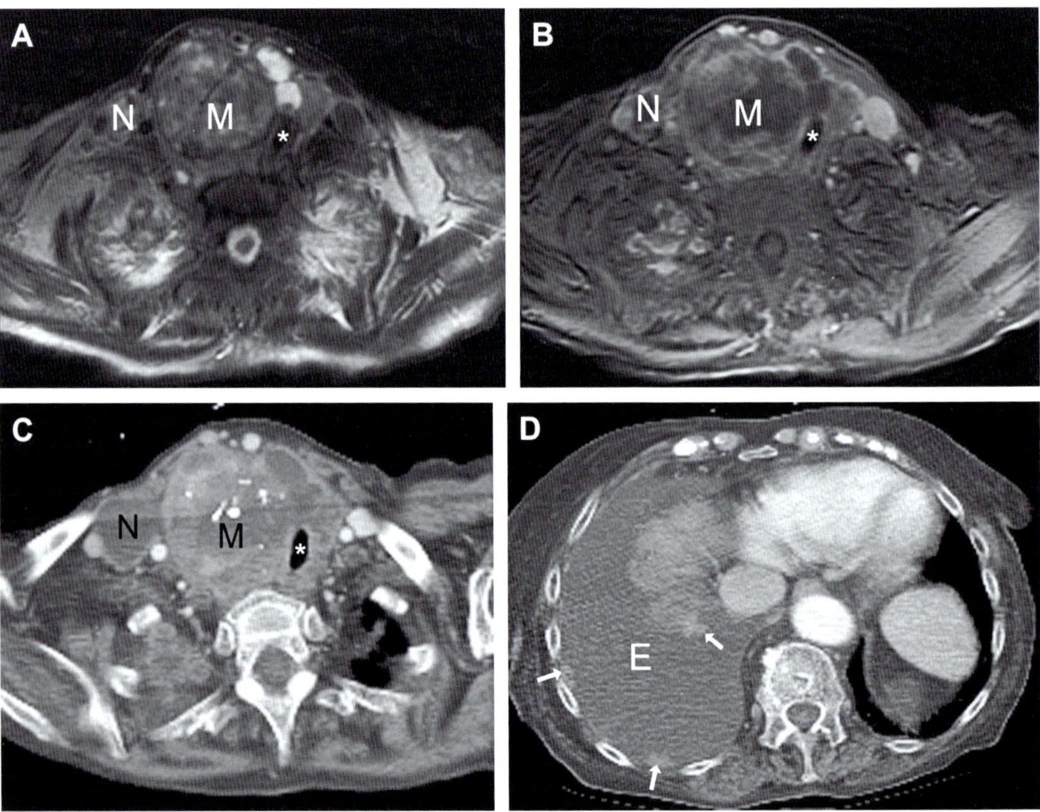

Fig. 6. Seventy-nine-year-old woman with chronic multinodular goiter presents with new right cervical mass, hoarseness, and right upper extremity weakness due to poorly differentiated metastatic thyroid carcinoma. Axial T2-W (*A*) and contrast-enhanced fat-suppressed T1-W (*B*) MR images and axial contrast-enhanced CT image (*C*) through neck demonstrate large mass (M) of thyroid gland with heterogeneous SI, attenuation, and enhancement with associated leftward deviation and moderate narrowing of tracheal lumen (*asterisks*) as well as regional necrotic lymphadenopathy (N). (*D*) Axial contrast-enhanced CT image through lower thorax shows large right pleural effusion (E) with pleural soft tissue nodules (*arrows*) due to metastatic disease.

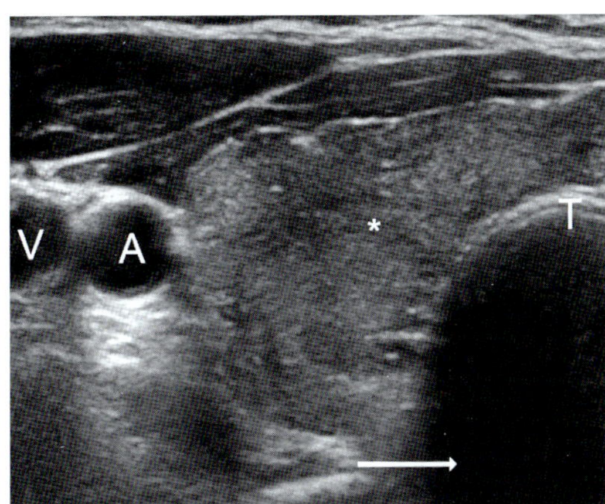

Fig. 7. Forty-six-year-old man with goiter due to chronic lymphocytic thyroiditis. Axial gray-scale ultrasound image through thyroid gland shows diffusely enlarged thyroid gland (*asterisk*) with heterogeneous predominantly hypoechoic echotexture. Note anechoic internal carotid artery (A) and internal jugular vein (V) as well as posterior acoustic shadowing (*arrow*) due to poor transmission of sound waves through trachea (T).

generally is not administered to patients if such diagnostic and therapeutic nuclear medicine techniques are anticipated in the near future.[42]

CT, MR imaging, and ultrasonography can also reveal diffuse enlargement of the thyroid gland either incidentally or in patients specifically referred for structural imaging evaluation of a mediastinal or neck mass detected on physical examination or other imaging modality. The major differential diagnostic considerations for thyroid enlargement include a multinodular goiter and Graves' disease. The diffusely enlarged thyroid gland may have either homogeneous or heterogeneous attenuation,

SI, and echogenicity, and may have a smooth or nodular contour (**Fig. 7**).[40,41,43] Sometimes, when the thyroid gland becomes markedly enlarged, portions of the gland can extend into the anterior or middle mediastinum and exert mass effect on or cause luminal compromise of adjacent structures, such as the trachea and great vessels (**Fig. 8**).[44] In Graves' disease, intense hypervascularity is a characteristic finding on color Doppler ultrasound (**Fig. 9**).[45]

STRUCTURAL IMAGING OF THE ADRENAL GLANDS

CT and MR imaging are the structural imaging modalities most frequently used to evaluate the adrenal glands, whereas ultrasound is less frequently used because of its insensitivity for small lesions and frequent nonspecificity for characterization of detected adrenal abnormalities. The main clinical indications for CT and MR imaging evaluation of the adrenal glands are detection of macroscopic adrenal disease, such as in the setting of known malignancy or trauma, characterization of an indeterminate adrenal lesion detected either incidentally on prior imaging or during the staging workup for known malignancy, or for assessment of a suspected functional adrenal nodule or adrenal hyperplasia in the setting of known metabolic abnormality.[46,47]

In general, CT is used as the first-line imaging tool, whereas MR imaging is employed as a problem-solving tool (although it too can be used as the first-line imaging tool if there is a contraindication to performing a contrast-enhanced CT examination). If the structural imaging findings are nonspecific, then either follow-up imaging, positron emission tomography, or image-guided tissue

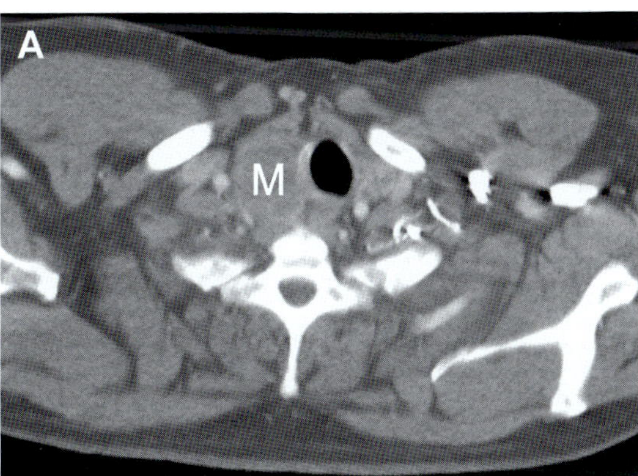

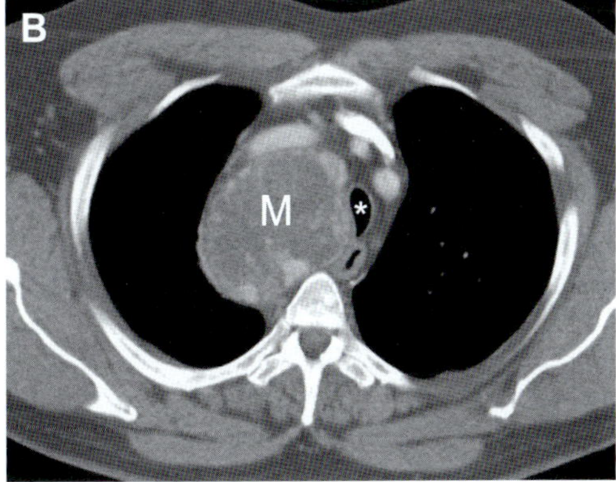

Fig. 8. Fifty-five-year-old man with mediastinal mass due to thyroid goiter. Axial contrast-enhanced CT images through neck (*A*) and upper thorax (*B*) reveal heterogeneously enhancing mass (M) arising from right lobe of thyroid gland with extension into middle mediastinum and associated leftward deviation and moderate narrowing of tracheal lumen (*asterisk*).

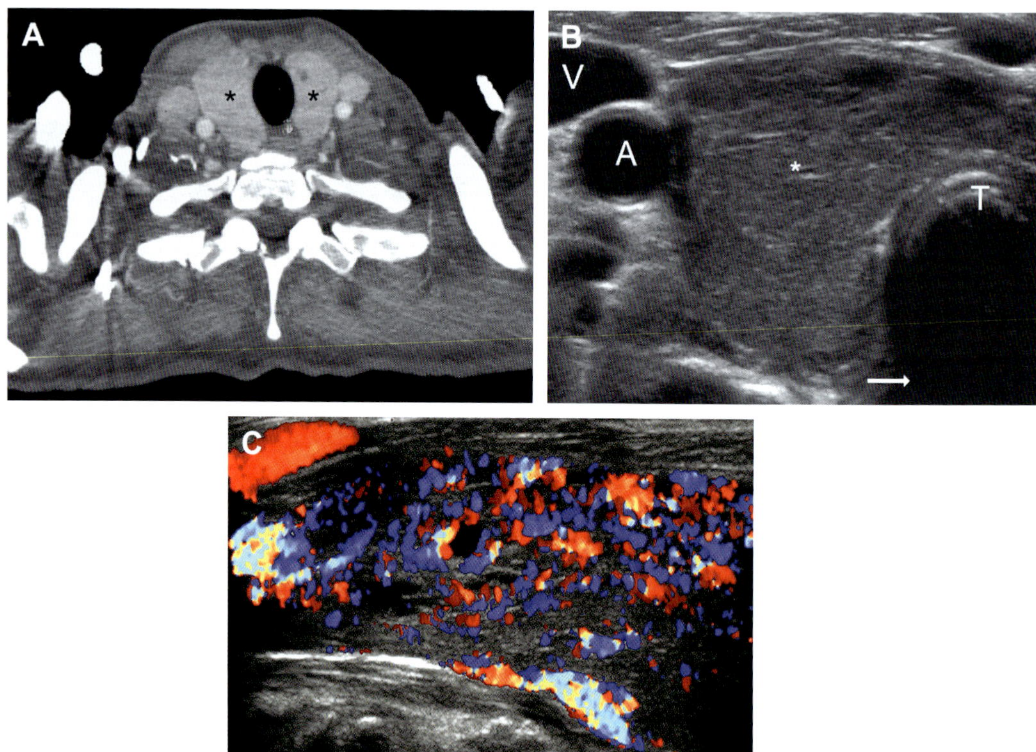

Fig. 9. Fifty-two-year-old woman with history of thyrotoxicosis and thyroid storm due to Graves' disease. (*A*) Axial contrast-enhanced CT image through neck demonstrates diffusely enlarged mildly heterogeneous thyroid gland (*asterisks*). Axial gray-scale (*B*) and sagittal color Doppler (*C*) images through right lobe of thyroid gland demonstrate diffuse gland enlargement with heterogeneous hypoechogenicity and intense hypervascularity. Note anechoic internal carotid artery (A) and internal jugular vein (V) as well as posterior acoustic shadowing (*arrow*) due to poor transmission of sound waves through trachea (T).

sampling is performed to obtain a more definitive diagnosis. CT and MR imaging are complementary with 18F-fluorodeoxyglucose positron emission tomography for evaluation of the adrenal glands, and together maximize the sensitivity, specificity, and accuracy of detection and characterization of adrenal lesions, particularly during the staging workup of patients with known malignancy.[1,48]

CT and MR imaging findings that are generally suggestive of a benign etiology for an adrenal lesion include small lesion size (<3 cm in diameter), a smooth margin, a decrease or no change in size over time, or diffuse enlargement of the adrenal gland with maintenance of adrenal shape, whereas imaging findings that are suggestive of a malignant etiology include large lesion size (especially when >5 cm in diameter), appearance of a new lesion or increase in lesion size over time, an irregular margin, heterogeneous attenuation or SI, invasion of surrounding tissues by the lesion, and other imaging findings of malignancy involving the remainder of the body, such as a visualization of a primary tumor, lymphadenopathy, or

hematogenous metastases.[47,49,50] A history of current or prior malignancy makes the possibility of an adrenal metastasis more likely as adrenal metastases are very common (occurring in

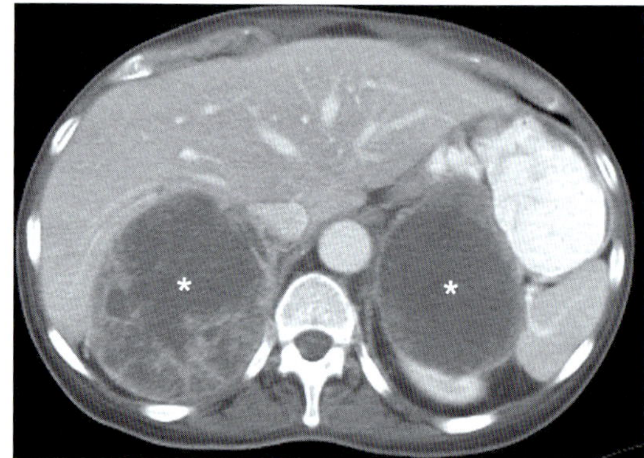

Fig. 10. Fifty-five-year-old woman with lung carcinoma with adrenal gland metastases. Axial contrast-enhanced CT image through upper abdomen demonstrates bilateral large heterogeneous cystic and solid enhancing adrenal gland masses (*asterisks*).

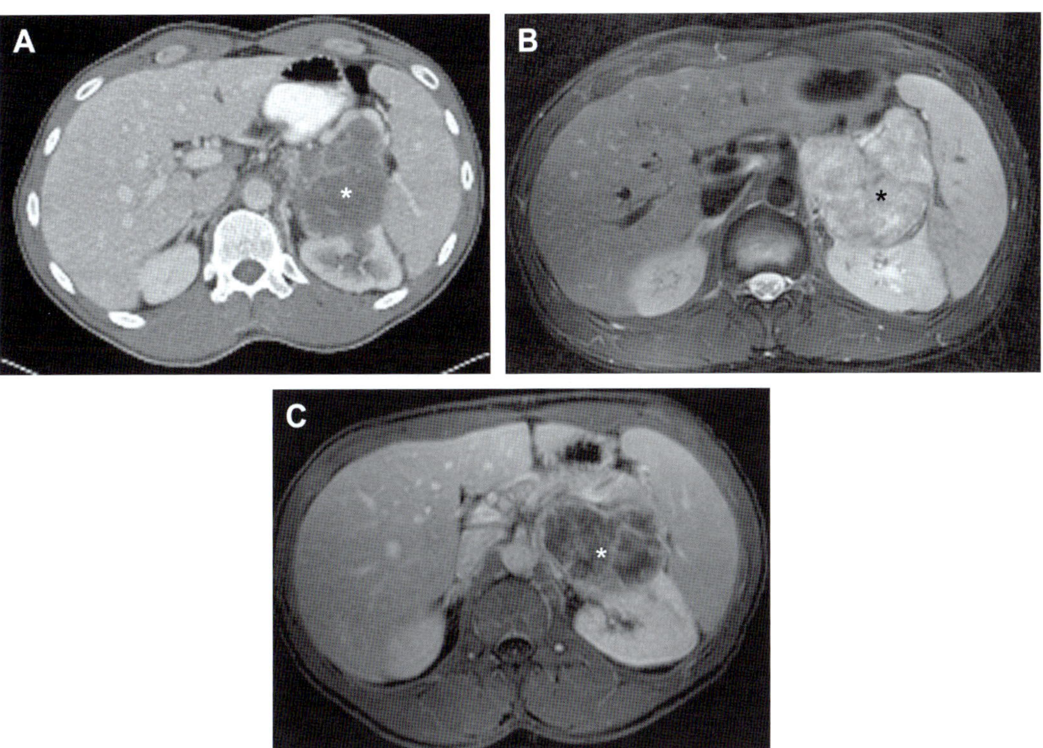

Fig. 11. Thirty-one-year-old man with poorly differentiated primary adrenocortical carcinoma. Axial contrast-enhanced CT (*A*), T2-W MR image (*B*), and contrast-enhanced fat-suppressed T1-W MR image (*C*) through upper abdomen show large heterogeneously enhancing mass (*asterisks*) centered in location of left adrenal gland. Metastatic disease to contralateral adrenal gland and retroperitoneal lymph nodes was also present (not shown).

approximately 25% of patients with epithelial malignancies at autopsy), most commonly in the setting of lung carcinoma, breast carcinoma, renal cell carcinoma, and melanoma (**Fig. 10**).[51,52] Primary adrenocortical carcinoma is a rare aggressive malignancy that should also be considered in the differential diagnosis of an adrenal lesion, particularly when a large heterogeneous unilateral adrenal mass, often in association with direct invasion of adjacent structures or distant metastatic disease, is seen on CT or MR image (**Fig. 11**).[52,53] Described below are additional imaging findings that are more specific for benign etiologies of adrenal disease.

The typical CT imaging protocol for evaluation of an indeterminate adrenal lesion involves acquisition of thin-section unenhanced images, contrast-enhanced images obtained soon after contrast administration during the parenchymal phase of enhancement, and delayed contrast-enhanced images obtained 10 to 20 minutes after contrast administration. On CT, some highly specific imaging findings for the diagnosis of an adrenal adenoma (the most common benign neoplasm of the adrenal gland) include an attenuation value on unenhanced CT of 10 or fewer Hounsfield

units (HU), an attenuation value of 37 or fewer HU on 15-minute delayed-phase contrast-enhanced images, or an absolute percentage washout (defined as [HU on contrast-enhanced parenchymal phase images − HU on 15-minute delayed-phase contrast-enhanced images]/[HU on contrast-enhanced parenchymal phase images − HU on unenhanced images] × 100%) or relative percentage washout (defined as [HU on contrast-enhanced parenchymal phase images − HU on 15-minute delayed-phase contrast-enhanced images]/[HU on contrast-enhanced parenchymal phase images] × 100%) of lesion enhancement of 60% or more or of 40% or more, respectively (**Fig. 12**).[54,55] On MR imaging, loss of SI on out-of-phase T1-W gradient-echo images relative to in-phase T1-W images within an adrenal lesion is specific for the diagnosis of an adrenal adenoma, as this finding reflects the presence of a mixture of intralesional microscopic lipid and water (**Fig. 13**).[56]

If atrophy of the contralateral adrenal gland is also visualized on CT or MR image, then a hypersecretory adrenal adenoma can be suggested. However, if contralateral adrenal gland atrophy is not detected, then one cannot determine whether an

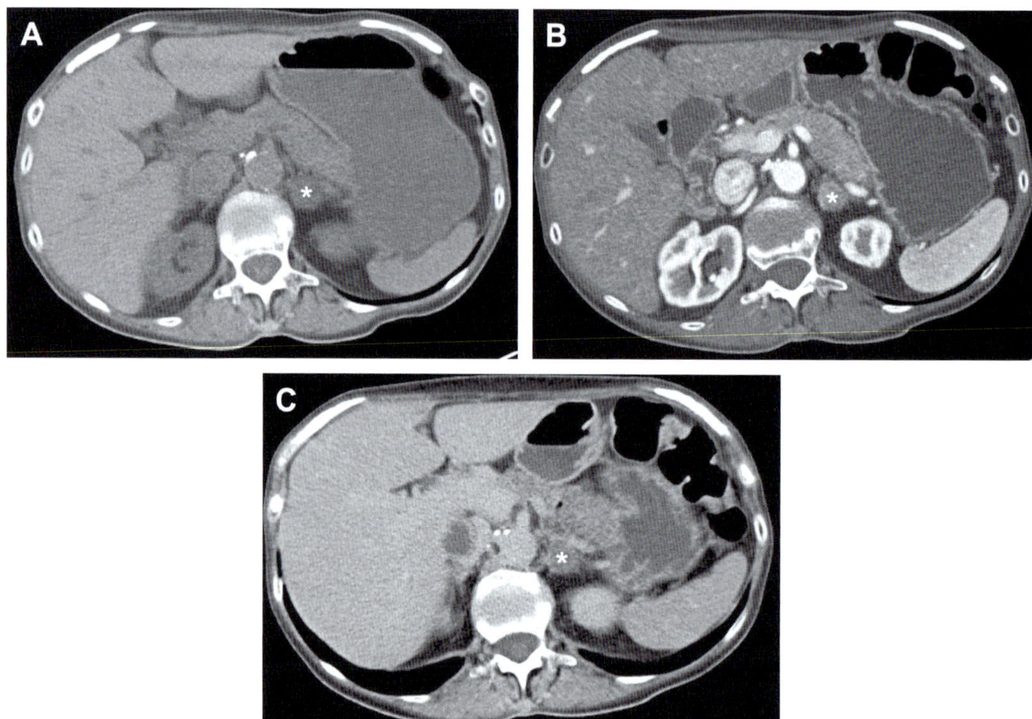

Fig. 12. Sixty-three-year-old woman with adrenal adenoma. (*A*) Axial unenhanced CT image through upper abdomen demonstrates 2-cm left adrenal gland nodule (*asterisk*) with attenuation of 10 HU, diagnostic for adrenal adenoma. Axial early parenchymal phase (*B*) and 15-minute delayed-phase contrast-enhanced (*C*) CT images at same location reveal nodule attenuation of 112 HU and 37 HU, respectively, with latter diagnostic for adrenal adenoma. Absolute percentage washout ([112 HU − 37 HU]/[112 HU − 10 HU] × 100%) is 74% (which is ≥ 60%) and relative percentage washout ([112 HU − 37 HU]/[112 HU] × 100%) is 67% (which is ≥ 40%), both diagnostic for adrenal adenoma as well.

adenoma is hypersecretory or nonhypersecretory on structural imaging alone. In this case, further evaluation with either adrenal vein sampling or nuclear scintigraphy may be indicated.[57]

The visualization of smooth diffuse enlargement of the adrenal glands on CT or MR image is suggestive of bilateral adrenal hyperplasia, particularly in the setting of known Conn's syndrome or

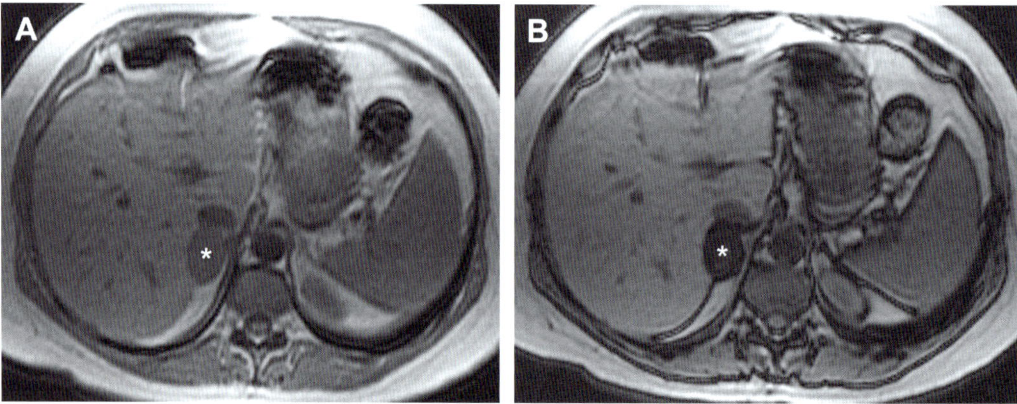

Fig. 13. Fifty-three-year-old woman with adrenal adenoma. Axial T1-W in-phase (*A*) and out-of-phase (*B*) gradient-echo images through upper abdomen show 3-cm well-circumscribed smoothly marginated right adrenal gland mass (*asterisks*) with intermediate SI relative to skeletal muscle on in-phase images and characteristic loss of SI on out-of-phase images indicative of presence of microscopic lipid within lesion. Note that only out-of-phase T1-W images demonstrate black etching artifacts where soft tissue organs and tissues contact high SI macroscopic fat in subcutaneous and visceral locations.

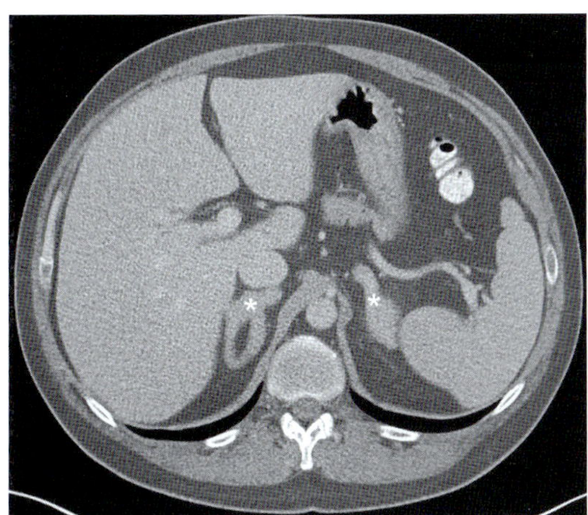

Fig. 14. Twenty-nine-year-old man with massive bilateral adrenal gland hyperplasia due to ectopic adrenocorticotropic hormone production by hilar neuroendocrine carcinoma. Axial contrast-enhanced CT image through upper abdomen reveals massive smooth diffuse enlargement of adrenal glands (*asterisks*).

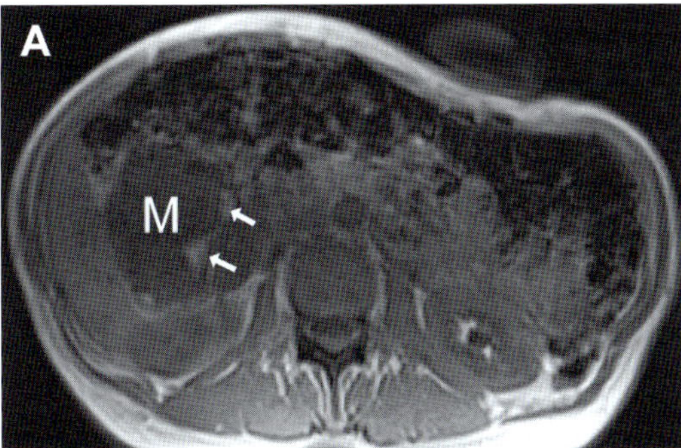

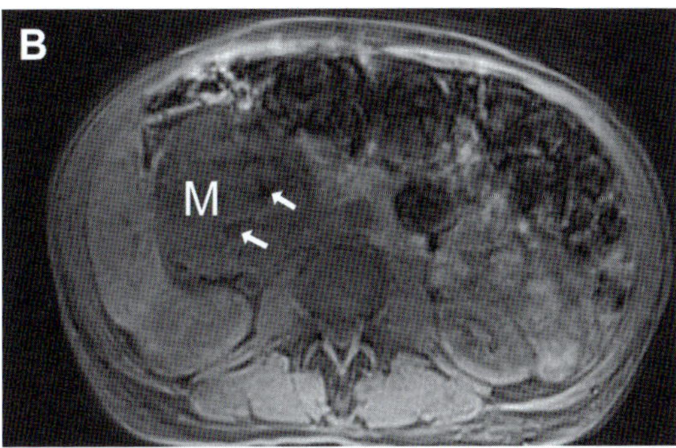

Fig. 15. Fifty-six-year-old woman with incidental adrenal myelolipoma. Axial T1-W MR images without (*A*) and with (*B*) fat suppression demonstrate 9-cm heterogeneous SI right adrenal mass (M) that contains foci of high T1-W SI that lose SI after fat suppression (*arrows*) indicative of macroscopic fat, diagnostic of adrenal myelolipoma. Note loss of SI of macroscopic fat elsewhere in subcutaneous and visceral compartments of abdomen after fat suppression.

Cushing's syndrome (**Fig. 14**). Differentiation of bilateral adrenal hyperplasia from a hypersecretory adrenal adenoma as the underlying cause of such conditions is important, as the former is treated medically and the latter is treated surgically. Adrenal vein sampling or nuclear scintigraphy may again be useful in cases where the CT or MR image findings are indeterminate or when no macroscopic adrenal gland abnormalities are detected despite the presence of metabolic abnormalities.[58–60]

Detection of macroscopic fat within an adrenal lesion on CT or MR image (with attenuation in the case of CT or SI in the case of MR image similar to that for subcutaneous fat) is diagnostic of an adrenal myelolipoma, which is a benign adrenal lesion composed of mature adipose cells and hematopoietic tissue (**Fig. 15**). A round or oval fluid

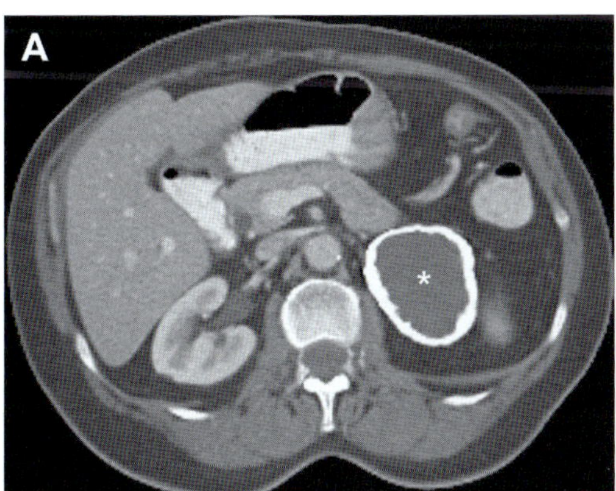

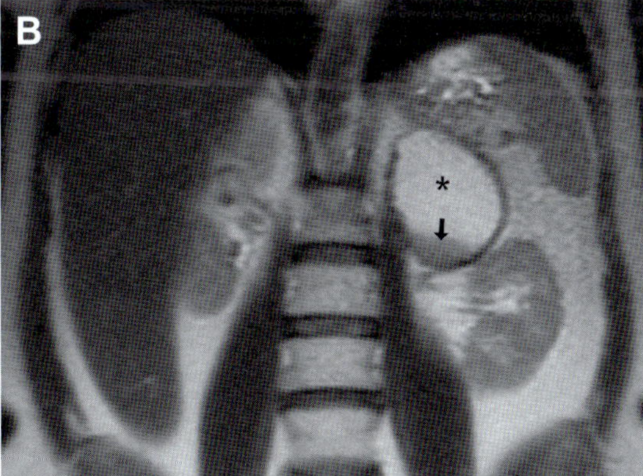

Fig. 16. Fifty-four-year-old woman with adrenal pseudocyst related to remote adrenal hematoma that occurred after anticoagulation therapy. (*A*) Axial contrast-enhanced CT image through upper abdomen shows 6-cm fluid attenuation lesion (*asterisk*) of left adrenal gland with very high attenuation rim calcification. (*B*) Coronal T2-W MR image through adrenal lesion demonstrates very high SI fluid within lesion (*asterisk*) with decreased SI inferiorly (*arrow*) due to proteinaceous debris. Note peripheral low SI rim due to fibrous tissue and calcification.

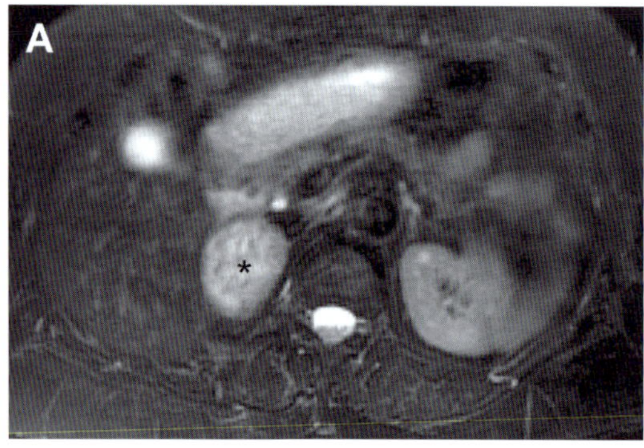

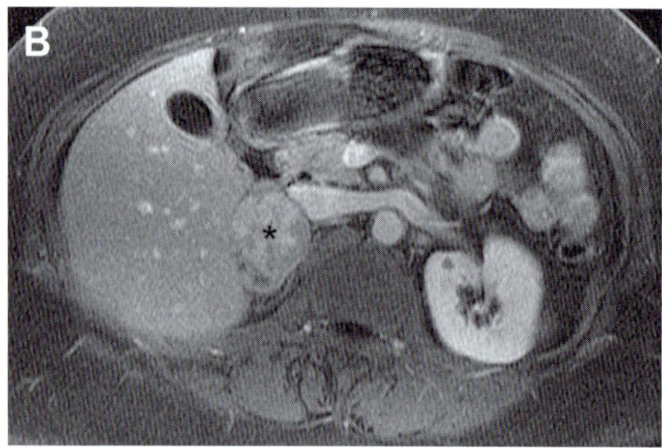

Fig. 17. Fifty-six-year-old woman with adrenal pheochromocytoma. (*A*) Axial fat-suppressed T2-W MR image through upper abdomen reveals 5-cm right adrenal mass (*asterisk*) with heterogeneously high SI relative to skeletal muscle. No microscopic lipid content was detected on T1-W gradient-echo images (not shown). (*B*) Axial contrast-enhanced fat-suppressed T1-W image through same level demonstrates avid enhancement of mass (*asterisk*).

attenuation or SI adrenal lesion with no solid enhancing components detected on CT or MR imaging is highly suggestive of an adrenal cyst or pseudocyst, particularly when very high attenuation rim calcification or an internal fluid-fluid level is encountered (**Fig. 16**).[61]

Pheochromocytomas are rare catecholamine-secreting tumors that characteristically appear as hypervascular adrenal masses on contrast-enhanced CT and MR image often with areas of low attenuation or high T2-W SI but without microscopic lipid on T1-W gradient-echo images (**Fig. 17**). However, fatty, hemorrhagic, cystic, or calcific changes may be encountered, making this specific diagnosis more difficult to make on structural imaging alone.[62,63] Ten percent of pheochromocytomas are malignant, but the only structural imaging definitive finding of a malignant pheochromocytoma is that of metastatic disease elsewhere in the body.[62] Laboratory assessment of the urine for the presence of catecholamine metabolites can be very useful to make a more definitive diagnosis of adrenal pheochromocytoma.[64]

SUMMARY

CT, MR imaging, and ultrasonography each play an important role in the clinical management of patients with disease conditions of the endocrine system, and are complementary with functional and molecular imaging techniques. As such, it is important for the nuclear medicine physician and radiologist to be aware of the overall and organ-specific advantages and disadvantages of employing these modalities, and to have an understanding of the basic imaging manifestations of disease entities that may affect the endocrine system.

REFERENCES

1. Torigian DA, Huang SS, Houseni M, et al. Functional imaging of cancer with emphasis on molecular techniques. CA Cancer J Clin 2007;57(4):206–24.
2. Rydberg J, Liang Y, Teague SD. Fundamentals of multichannel CT. Radiol Clin North Am 2003;41(3): 465–74.
3. Nikken JJ, Krestin GP. MRI of the kidney—state of the art. Eur Radiol 2007;17(11):2780–93.
4. Kanal E, Barkovich AJ, Bell C, et al. ACR guidance document for safe MR practices: 2007. AJR Am J Roentgenol 2007;188(6):1447–74.
5. Brenner DJ, Hall EJ. Computed tomography—an increasing source of radiation exposure. N Engl J Med 2007;357(22):2277–84.
6. Thomsen HS. European Society of Urogenital Radiology (ESUR) guidelines on the safe use of iodinated contrast media. Eur J Radiol 2006;60(3):307–13.
7. Perazella MA, Rodby RA. Gadolinium use in patients with kidney disease: a cause for concern. Semin Dial 2007;20(3):179–85.
8. Hangiandreou NJ. AAPM/RSNA physics tutorial for residents. Topics in US: B-mode US: basic concepts and new technology. Radiographics 2003;23(4): 1019–33.
9. Miki Y, Kanagaki M, Takahashi JA, et al. Evaluation of pituitary macroadenomas with multidetector-row CT (MDCT): comparison with MR imaging. Neuroradiology 2007;49(4):327–33.
10. Elster AD. Modern imaging of the pituitary. Radiology 1993;187(1):1–14.
11. Steiner E, Knosp E, Herold CJ, et al. Pituitary adenomas: findings of postoperative MR imaging. Radiology 1992;185(2):521–7.
12. Pierallini A, Caramia F, Falcone C, et al. Pituitary macroadenomas: preoperative evaluation of consistency with diffusion-weighted MR imaging—initial experience. Radiology 2006;239(1):223–31.
13. Gsponer J, De Tribolet N, Deruaz JP, et al. Diagnosis, treatment, and outcome of pituitary tumors and other abnormal intrasellar masses. Retrospective

analysis of 353 patients. Medicine (Baltimore) 1999; 78(4):236–69.

14. Saeger W, Ludecke DK, Buchfelder M, et al. Pathohistological classification of pituitary tumors: 10 years of experience with the German Pituitary Tumor Registry. Eur J Endocrinol 2007;156(2):203–16.

15. Tosaka M, Sato N, Hirato J, et al. Assessment of hemorrhage in pituitary macroadenoma by T2*-weighted gradient-echo MR imaging. AJNR Am J Neuroradiol 2007;28(10):2023–9.

16. Miki Y, Matsuo M, Nishizawa S, et al. Pituitary adenomas and normal pituitary tissue: enhancement patterns on gadopentetate-enhanced MR imaging. Radiology 1990;177(1):35–8.

17. Sakamoto Y, Takahashi M, Korogi Y, et al. Normal and abnormal pituitary glands: gadopentetate dimeglumine-enhanced MR imaging. Radiology 1991;178(2):441–5.

18. Barkan AL. Pituitary atrophy in patients with Sheehan's syndrome. Am J Med Sci 1989;298(1):38–40.

19. Thodou E, Asa SL, Kontogeorgos G, et al. Clinical case seminar: lymphocytic hypophysitis: clinicopathological findings. J Clin Endocrinol Metab 1995;80(8):2302–11.

20. Shimono T, Hatabu H, Kasagi K, et al. Rapid progression of pituitary hyperplasia in humans with primary hypothyroidism: demonstration with MR imaging. Radiology 1999;213(2):383–8.

21. Giustina A, Gola M, Doga M, et al. Clinical review 136: Primary lymphoma of the pituitary: an emerging clinical entity. J Clin Endocrinol Metab 2001;86(10): 4567–75.

22. Vates GE, Berger MS, Wilson CB. Diagnosis and management of pituitary abscess: a review of twenty-four cases. J Neurosurg 2001;95(2):233–41.

23. Ragel BT, Couldwell WT. Pituitary carcinoma: a review of the literature. Neurosurg Focus 2004; 16(4):E7.

24. Fassett DR, Couldwell WT. Metastases to the pituitary gland. Neurosurg Focus 2004;16(4):E8.

25. Hall WA, Luciano MG, Doppman JL, et al. Pituitary magnetic resonance imaging in normal human volunteers: occult adenomas in the general population. Ann Intern Med 1994;120(10):817–20.

26. King JT Jr, Justice AC, Aron DC. Management of incidental pituitary microadenomas: a cost-effectiveness analysis. J Clin Endocrinol Metab 1997;82(11):3625–32.

27. Mortensen JD, Woolner LB, Bennett WA. Gross and microscopic findings in clinically normal thyroid glands. J Clin Endocrinol Metab 1955;15(10): 1270–80.

28. Brander A, Viikinkoski P, Nickels J, et al. Thyroid gland: US screening in a random adult population. Radiology 1991;181(3):683–7.

29. Bruneton JN, Balu-Maestro C, Marcy PY, et al. Very high frequency (13 MHz) ultrasonographic examination of the normal neck: detection of normal lymph nodes and thyroid nodules. J Ultrasound Med 1994;13(2):87–90.

30. Wiest PW, Hartshorne MF, Inskip PD, et al. Thyroid palpation versus high-resolution thyroid ultrasonography in the detection of nodules. J Ultrasound Med 1998;17(8):487–96.

31. Frates MC, Benson CB, Charboneau JW, et al. Management of thyroid nodules detected at US: Society of Radiologists in Ultrasound consensus conference statement. Radiology 2005;237(3): 794–800.

32. Gilliland FD, Hunt WC, Morris DM, et al. Prognostic factors for thyroid carcinoma. A population-based study of 15,698 cases from the Surveillance, Epidemiology and End Results (SEER) program 1973–1991. Cancer 1997;79(3):564–73.

33. Jemal A, Siegel R, Ward E, et al. Cancer statistics, 2008. CA Cancer J Clin 2008;58(2):71–96.

34. Hoang JK, Lee WK, Lee M, et al. US Features of thyroid malignancy: pearls and pitfalls. Radiographics 2007;27(3):847–60 [discussion: 61–5].

35. Danese D, Sciacchitano S, Farsetti A, et al. Diagnostic accuracy of conventional versus sonography-guided fine-needle aspiration biopsy of thyroid nodules. Thyroid 1998;8(1):15–21.

36. Mittendorf EA, Tamarkin SW, McHenry CR. The results of ultrasound-guided fine-needle aspiration biopsy for evaluation of nodular thyroid disease. Surgery 2002;132(4):648–53 [discussion: 53–4].

37. Bellantone R, Lombardi CP, Raffaelli M, et al. Management of cystic or predominantly cystic thyroid nodules: the role of ultrasound-guided fine-needle aspiration biopsy. Thyroid 2004;14(1):43–7.

38. Gharib H, Papini E. Thyroid nodules: clinical importance, assessment, and treatment. Endocrinol Metab Clin North Am 2007;36(3):707–35, vi.

39. Johnson NA, Tublin ME, Ogilvie JB. Parathyroid imaging: technique and role in the preoperative evaluation of primary hyperparathyroidism. AJR Am J Roentgenol 2007;188(6):1706–15.

40. Weber AL, Randolph G, Aksoy FG. The thyroid and parathyroid glands. CT and MR imaging and correlation with pathology and clinical findings. Radiol Clin North Am 2000;38(5):1105–29.

41. Gotway MB, Higgins CB. MR imaging of the thyroid and parathyroid glands. Magn Reson Imaging Clin N Am 2000;8(1):163–82, ix.

42. van der Molen AJ, Thomsen HS, Morcos SK. Effect of iodinated contrast media on thyroid function in adults. Eur Radiol 2004;14(5):902–7.

43. Quint LE. Imaging of anterior mediastinal masses. Cancer Imaging 2007;(7 Spec No A):S56–62.

44. Strollo DC, Rosado de Christenson ML, Jett JR. Primary mediastinal tumors. Part 1: tumors of the anterior mediastinum. Chest 1997;112(2):511–22.

45. Erdogan MF, Anil C, Cesur M, et al. Color flow Doppler sonography for the etiologic diagnosis of hyperthyroidism. Thyroid 2007;17(3):223–8.

46. Mayo-Smith WW, Boland GW, Noto RB, et al. State-of-the-art adrenal imaging. Radiographics 2001; 21(4):995–1012.

47. Heinz-Peer G, Memarsadeghi M, Niederle B. Imaging of adrenal masses. Curr Opin Urol 2007;17(1): 32–8.

48. Alavi A, Lakhani P, Mavi A, et al. PET: a revolution in medical imaging. Radiol Clin North Am 2004;42(6): 983–1001, vii.

49. Siegelman ES. MR imaging of the adrenal neoplasms. Magn Reson Imaging Clin N Am 2000; 8(4):769–86.

50. Caoili EM, Korobkin M, Francis IR, et al. Adrenal masses: characterization with combined unenhanced and delayed enhanced CT. Radiology 2002;222(3):629–33.

51. Abrams HL, Spiro R, Goldstein N. Metastases in carcinoma; analysis of 1000 autopsied cases. Cancer 1950;3(1):74–85.

52. Fassnacht M, Kenn W, Allolio B. Adrenal tumors: how to establish malignancy? J Endocrinol Invest 2004;27(4):387–99.

53. Ng L, Libertino JM. Adrenocortical carcinoma: diagnosis, evaluation and treatment. J Urol 2003; 169(1):5–11.

54. Korobkin M, Brodeur FJ, Francis IR, et al. CT time-attenuation washout curves of adrenal adenomas and nonadenomas. AJR Am J Roentgenol 1998; 170(3):747–52.

55. Caoili EM, Korobkin M, Francis IR, et al. Delayed enhanced CT of lipid-poor adrenal adenomas. AJR Am J Roentgenol 2000;175(5):1411–5.

56. Outwater EK, Siegelman ES, Radecki PD, et al. Distinction between benign and malignant adrenal masses: value of T1-weighted chemical-shift MR imaging. AJR Am J Roentgenol 1995;165(3): 579–83.

57. Choyke PL, Doppman JL. Case 18: adrenocorticotropic hormone-dependent Cushing syndrome. Radiology 2000;214(1):195–8.

58. Doppman JL, Gill JR Jr, Miller DL, et al. Distinction between hyperaldosteronism due to bilateral hyperplasia and unilateral aldosteronoma: reliability of CT. Radiology 1992;184(3):677–82.

59. Phillips JL, Walther MM, Pezzullo JC, et al. Predictive value of preoperative tests in discriminating bilateral adrenal hyperplasia from an aldosterone-producing adrenal adenoma. J Clin Endocrinol Metab 2000; 85(12):4526–33.

60. Patel SM, Lingam RK, Beaconsfield TI, et al. Role of radiology in the management of primary aldosteronism. Radiographics 2007;27(4):1145–57.

61. Sahdev A, Reznek RH. The indeterminate adrenal mass in patients with cancer. Cancer Imaging 2007;(7 Spec No A):S100–9.

62. Blake MA, Kalra MK, Maher MM, et al. Pheochromocytoma: an imaging chameleon. Radiographics 2004;24(Suppl 1):S87–99.

63. Andreoni C, Krebs RK, Bruna PC, et al. Cystic phaeochromocytoma is a distinctive subgroup with special clinical, imaging and histological features that might mislead the diagnosis. BJU Int 2007;101(3):345–50.

64. Zelinka T, Eisenhofer G, Pacak K. Pheochromocytoma as a catecholamine producing tumor: implications for clinical practice. Stress 2007;10(2): 195–203.

Index

Note: Page numbers of article titles are in **boldface** type.

PET Clin 2 (2008) 409–411
doi:10.1016/S1556-8598(08)00049-7

Moving?

Make sure your subscription moves with you!

To notify us of your new address, find your **Clinics Account Number** (located on your mailing label above your name), and contact customer service at:

E-mail: elspcs@elsevier.com

800-654-2452 (subscribers in the U.S. & Canada)
1-407-563-6020 (subscribers outside of the U.S. & Canada)

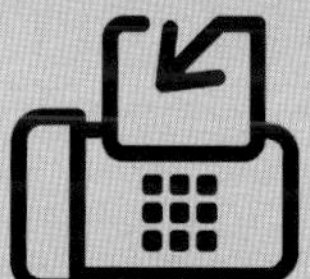

Fax number: 407-363-9661

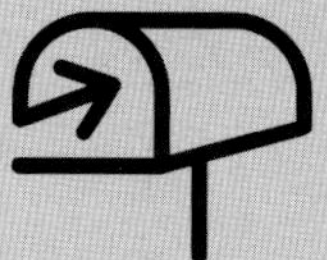

Elsevier Periodicals Customer Service
6277 Sea Harbor Drive
Orlando, FL 32887-4800

*To ensure uninterrupted delivery of your subscription, please notify us at least 4 weeks in advance of move.

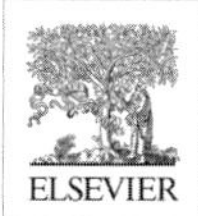